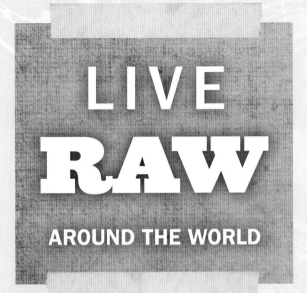

LIVE
RAW
AROUND THE WORLD

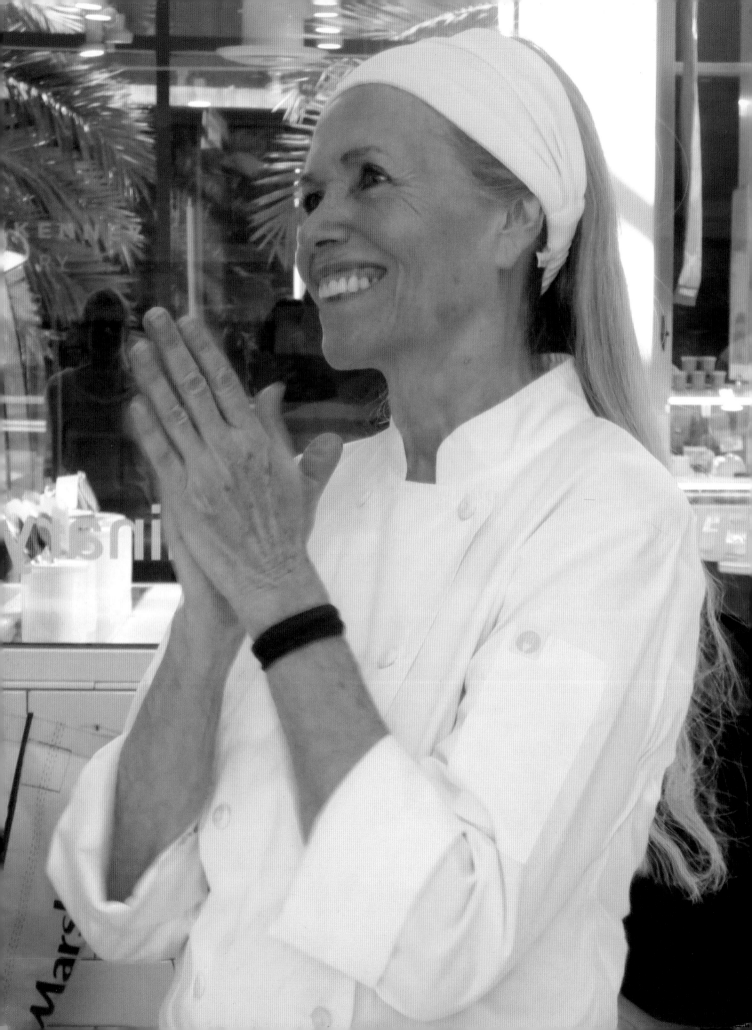

LIVE RAW

AROUND THE WORLD
International Raw Food Recipes for Good Health and Timeless Beauty

Mimi Kirk

Photography by
Mike Mendell

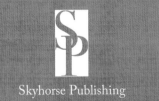

Skyhorse Publishing

Skyhorse Publishing books may be purchased in bulk at special discounts for sales promotion, corporate gifts, fund-raising, or educational purposes. Special editions can also be created to specifications. For details, contact the Special Sales Department, Skyhorse Publishing, 307 West 36th Street, 11th Floor, New York, NY 10018 or info@skyhorsepublishing.com.

Skyhorse® and Skyhorse Publishing® are registered trademarks of Skyhorse Publishing, Inc.®, a Delaware corporation.

www.skyhorsepublishing.com

10 9 8 7 6 5 4 3 2 1

Library of Congress Cataloging-in-Publication Data is available on file.

ISBN: 987-1-62087-613-8

Printed in China

"Twenty years from now you will be more disappointed by the things that you didn't do than by the ones you did do. So throw off the bowlines. Sail away from the safe harbor. Catch the trade winds in your sails. Explore. Dream. Discover."

~ Mark Twain

ABOUT THE AUTHOR

I'm a septuagenarian born in 1938. I am grateful for my outlook on life today. I like sharing what I've experienced to help others recognize that age is not a barrier to enjoying life. Anything can happen. A surprise turn in one's life can take place at any age.

For example, I completely changed to a raw vegan diet at the age of sixty-nine, and in September 2009, one week before my seventy-first birthday, I won the title "Sexiest Vegetarian over 50" in a nationwide contest conducted by PETA, People for the Ethical Treatment of Animals.

This title put me in the public eye and on the covers of magazines around the world, including Bulgaria, Portugal, Australia, Germany, and the U.K. I've appeared numerous times on national television in the United States and have been interviewed by major television and radio stations, newspapers, webinars, and Internet blogs. I was featured on Bulgarian and German television and appear in an Australian documentary titled *Eternal Youth*, to be released this year.

MY HOLLYWOOD DAYS

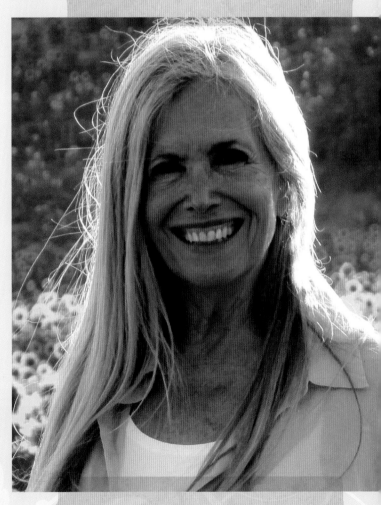

I was born in Hollywood, California, the youngest of seven children. I was married at seventeen and widowed at twenty-nine; I am the mother of two girls and two boys and a grandmother of seven grandchildren. After being a stay-at-home mother, I immediately had to find a job to support my family as there was no insurance or bank account after my husband's death. Fortunately, I was lucky enough to find a job as a screen extra in the film industry.

I worked in numerous television shows and movies. You might have seen me offering Captain Kirk a tray of fruit in an episode of the original *Star Trek*, in which I played an Indian handmaiden, or walking an ape on a leash in *Planet of the Apes*, or if you didn't blink, you might have seen me sitting at a table with Red Buttons and Shelley Winters in the original *Poseidon Adventure*, where I eventually jumped (or supposedly was tossed) over a railing as the boat was sinking.

In 1970, Mary Tyler Moore hired me to be her stand-in on her new sitcom, *The Mary Tyler Moore Show*. I also worked with Valerie Harper, designing and creating a good deal of her wardrobe, including the famous headscarf she wore in *Rhoda*. Throughout my entertainment career of eighteen years, I appeared in front of the camera as well as behind the scenes.

FINDING MY SPIRITUAL PATH

In 1968, shortly after my husband's death, I found my spiritual path. Meditation gave me strength and knowledge and taught me about the ebb and flow of life. It inspired me to live more in the moment and enjoy everything that each day had to offer. I was blessed to study with two living gurus: Swami Prabhavananda of the Vedanta Society and, later, after Swami Prabhavananda's death in 1976, Swami Muktananda of Siddah Yoga.

In 1983, shortly after Swami Muktananda's passing, I traveled to Ganeshpuri, India, and studied in my guru's ashram with his successor, a woman known as Gurumayi, or Swami Chidvilasananda.

In her 2006 book *Eat, Pray, Love*, Elizabeth Gilbert mentions she lived in an ashram for a short time. It was the same ashram I studied in years before, and just reading her words took me back to my own life-changing experiences. I also reminisce every time I see the movie.

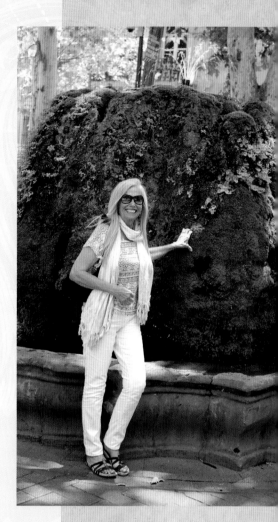

CAREER MOVES

A short time after returning from India, I decided to leave the film industry and try my hand at being entrepreneurial. I started a jewelry company and designed and manufactured costume jewelry sold to stores around the country.

After selling my company, I took a job in a private home in Beverly Hills as majordomo for a wealthy family. I oversaw all aspects of their estate and helped to create and implement charitable events. My environmental concerns became very strong, and after three years I left my job to create, publish, and edit *The City Planet*, an environmental newspaper in Los Angeles. I later moved to Taos, New Mexico, to find the "simple life," and while there, I helped start the city's first film festival.

In 1998, I created the first board game specifically geared toward women, titled *Cowgirls Ride the Trail of Truth*, and in 2000, I authored my first book, *Cowgirl Spirit*.

This is only a small part of my many incarnations, including a short stint as a Las Vegas showgirl at the Flamingo Hotel in 1957.

CURRENTLY

I manage my social networks and make YouTube videos on how to prepare raw foods. I write, research, and wander around my tiny kitchen creating new raw food recipes.

I walk almost every day, do some yoga, tend my garden, travel with my boyfriend, and spend time with my family. I give plant-based food demonstrations, coach clients, and consult. All this activity is something I would have never expected to be part of my life in my seventies, and this experience has taught me that anything is possible at any age.

www.youngonrawfood.com
www.facebook.com/pages/Mimi-Kirk/109888045694543
https://twitter.com/mimikirk

contents

INTRODUCTION   1

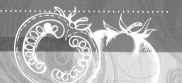

CHAPTER 13

RAW CUISINE – TASTE OF GERMANY   115

CHAPTER 14

RAW CUISINE – TASTE OF ITALY   133

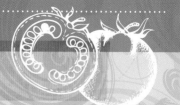

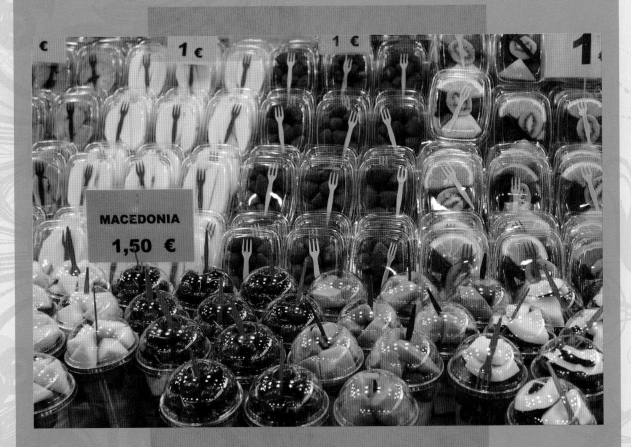

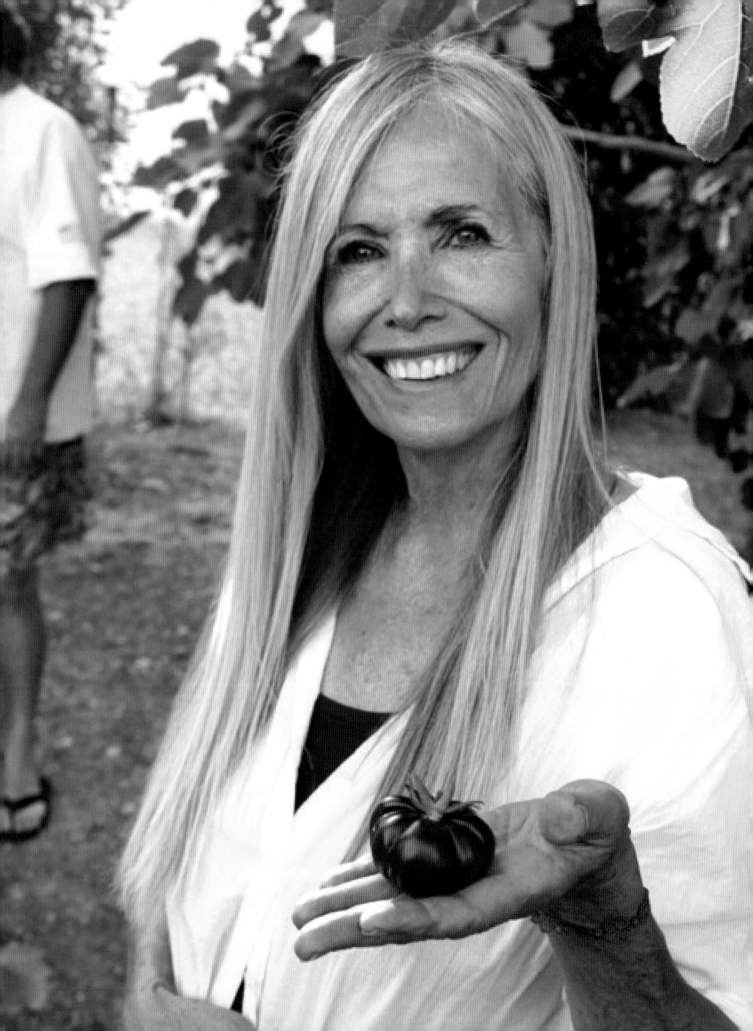

INTRODUCTION

The handwriting was on the wall. I was sixty-nine. My doctor told me I was just getting older and "things" are to be expected. "A few small pills daily could solve the problems," he said. Those "things" he was referring to were high blood pressure, high cholesterol, arthritis, and an extra twenty pounds.

That was all I needed to hear. I knew something would have to change or I would be living on medication for the rest of my life. When I returned home from my doctor's appointment, I opened my computer and started to research. I knew there must be some way to cure my ills naturally, without drugs.

I wondered why a raw food diet kept showing up in my searches. How could I look forward to enjoying life by eating carrots and celery? I'm a foodie who loves to cook—and I love to eat even more.

I thought I was a healthy eater, at least compared with most people I knew.

I'd been a vegetarian/vegan for the better part of forty years and never thought there was any better way to eat. The longer I researched, however, the more I learned. Testimonials claimed that eating a raw food diet cured many illnesses and diseases. Many had lost hundreds of pounds and gained more energy and stamina. I was definitely intrigued.

Many raw foodists put into practice what's called a detox. They claim that drinking juices and eating salads release toxins from the body naturally. I decided to try it for one week. To my surprise, I felt a positive difference in just a few days. When the week was over, I had lost weight and felt energized. I wanted more.

Making the decision to continue eating raw foods, I spent more hours researching and experimenting with different recipes. I was fascinated. The food tasted really good, and in no time, using recipes I had found as well as a few of my own creations, I was hooked on the challenge and technique of making raw food. I learned that to preserve the enzymes that aid in digestion, food must not be heated over 115° F.

I knew that if was going to continue eating this way, I would have to learn to prepare raw foods that would satisfy my taste buds on a daily basis. I would also need to satisfy my cravings for cooked foods. Most dishes I made turned out pretty fantastic; others went into the compost pile, the trash, or down the drain.

My taste buds started to change, and so did my digestion. I became addicted to morning green drinks. Cooked food I used to eat made my stomach feel bloated. I could feel and see the difference between eating cooked food versus raw food.

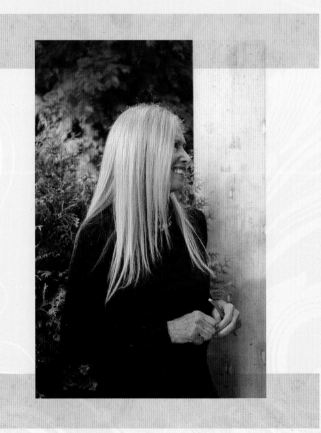

Sometimes it was more work than at other times, but I just kept feeling younger and healthier, so I couldn't stop. It took about a year of experimentation before it became easy to prepare a variety of dishes I loved.

Throughout that first year, my cravings started to diminish. I became more in touch with my body. It was telling me what I needed to eat, and I was listening. My twenty extra pounds dropped away quickly and never came back. My high blood pressure, cholesterol, and arthritis became a thing of the past. I was experiencing how raw food could allow me to live a longer, healthier life, and I knew I was onto something exciting. Giving up a few foods I used to enjoy in exchange for the vitality and health I currently experience was a small price to pay.

I appreciate how blessed I am to be healthy and to have gained the knowledge to stay healthy. At my age, I know that life without good health can be difficult.

Many men and women focus on how they look rather than how they feel. Trying to improve our appearance and look younger in unnatural ways using Botox injections, plastic surgery, and other artificial procedures can cause health risks. The results of procedures can turn out looking stiff and unnatural. There is no return from a "bad job" except to have more plastic surgery. There is no point in having perfect breasts, an unlined face, or a flat stomach if you are not in good health. I personally don't mind my character lines; in fact, I embrace each decade of change. I'm more concerned about staying healthy.

There is no need to stop dreaming and having goals as we age. The thrill of watching our children grow up, our grandchildren become parents, and maybe being around to play with our great-great-grandchildren is reason enough to want to stay healthy.

I plan on accomplishing more, having new experiences, and trying new things. I don't think about what I can't do at my age; I think about what I can do. I continue to see myself as a work in progress.

I am grateful to have a positive outlook, which has enabled me to get pleasure from an interesting and colorful life. Like most of us, I've had my share of ups and downs, joys and heartaches. I was married as a young girl of seventeen, a widow at twenty-nine, a single mom, a businesswoman, an entrepreneur, and after my children were grown, I was married and divorced, I became a single woman again. I can relate to women in many stages of life.

Many people retire or reach the age of fifty and think their best days are in the past. But with good health, self-love, and a positive attitude, exciting experiences can take place regardless of age. For example, I prepare delicious raw food, but I've always wanted to be a chef, not just a cook, so in February 2013 I completed a raw and living foods chef course at Matthew Kenney Culinary Academy, a state-of-the-art raw food culinary school adjacent to his restaurant M.A.K.E. in Santa Monica, California. In my mid-seventies, I am now an accredited, classically trained raw food chef.

My life is very fulfilling. My family is most important to me. I have a very close relationship with my children and grandchildren. I'm in a wonderful long-term relationship with my boyfriend, Mike, who is almost twenty years my junior, and life is good.

"Your regrets aren't what you did, but what you didn't do. So I take every opportunity."

~ Cameron Diaz

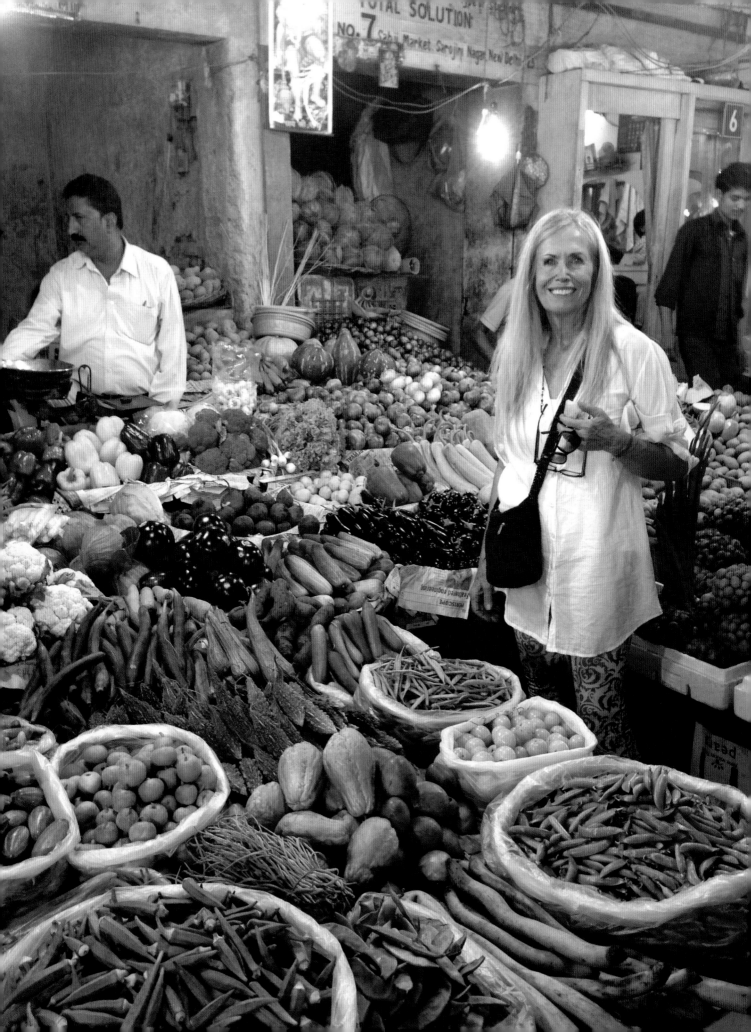

CHAPTER 1

· ·

THE MAKING OF LIVE RAW AROUND THE

WORLD

· ·

how it all started

Since my first cook book *Live Raw* was successful, my publishers asked me to write another raw food recipe book. I was still quite happy and enjoying meeting so many nice people through *Live Raw* and hadn't thought about writing another book. However, I'm a believer that if an opportunity comes your way, carpe diem (seize the day).

Once the idea of writing another raw food book sunk in, my creative mind just took over and I quickly came up with an idea that seemed exciting. I checked in with Mike, since he is involved in everything I do, and he thought it was a great idea, too. My idea was to combine our passion for travel and my love for international food, and *Live Raw Around the World* came to life.

This is not just a book of recipes. I hope to accomplish several things with *Live Raw Around the World*. One is to encourage women and men to enjoy life every day. Time really does go by quickly. I hear many people say, "I'd love to take a trip, but when this or that happens, then I'll go." Or, "I'll change my diet or start to exercise when I have more time." It takes planning, saving, and organization to travel. It takes commitment to diet and exercise. Although it might take effort for these things to happen, the outcome will be well worth it because of the happiness it brings.

Taking risks, staying positive, and being open to change helped me grow as a person in so many ways. I grew up in a lower-middle-class family that lived a very simple life. My siblings and I were not encouraged to go to college, as neither of our parents had completed high school. College was never mentioned in our house. We were never encouraged to have a particular career path besides my mother telling me to learn to type and write in shorthand so I could be a secretary in case I didn't marry. We rarely ate out in restaurants, and we lived in a tiny two-bedroom home where the kitchen stove was also used to heat the house.

Having grown up in this environment and having moved on to realize so many of my dreams, I offer you this advice: Follow your heart, and create a life that brings you health and happiness. Don't let your past dictate your future. Only you can make yourself happy. It's not someone else's responsibility. Only you decide what passes your lips, both incoming by what you eat and outgoing by what you say. Only you decide if you think either positive or negative thoughts.

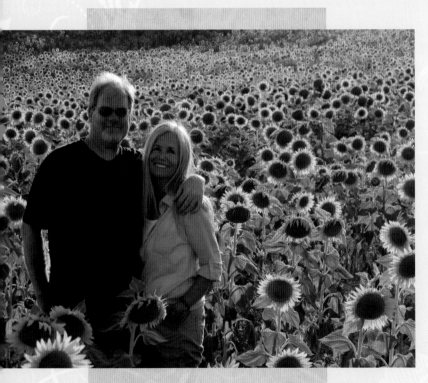

Improving your health is important to me, and throughout the book I've included many findings on the subject of processed food, factory farming, proteins, organic food, and how to live a longer, healthier life. The more you know, the better choices you will make for yourself and your family's health.

I could have written *Live Raw Around the World* with my current knowledge of international foods without ever leaving home, or I could make the choice to travel, visit each country, and create a new, fresh, authentic, and exciting book. Of course I chose the latter. My creative juices became amped up and started working overtime. My thoughts from that point on for many months seemed to be focused solely on the new book. Obsession? Maybe!

Thanks to Mike's diligent work on finding economical flights and deals on accommodations, and after many hours of booking, we were able to travel to many countries. We visited restaurants, private homes, farms, streets, and alleyways to absorb the local flavors. We searched for organic fruits, vegetables, herbs, and spices at neighborhood market places. We talked to farmers and asked what their growing methods involved, being particularly interested in whether or not they used chemical sprays. We learned how passionate many of them were about the produce they grew and sold, and their concerns about the land and future soil conditions. Everywhere we traveled, people were concerned about genetically modified food and seeds. We spoke with locals to find out more about meals they prepared at home, and we searched high and low to meet as many raw foodists and vegans in every country we visited.

With broken Italian, French, and Spanish, we worked our way through each country with our dictionaries and iPhone translator app. I knew from all my previous travels that a smile goes a long way and laughter is a universal language. The two together became our most prized communication skill. We connected with hundreds of people, made many new friends, and learned a few new words and a few more broken dialects. We had the most remarkable, informative, productive, and fun trip we could have ever imagined.

traveling companions

What would a recipe book be without photos to entice us? When I mention "we" in the chapters to follow, I'm talking about my partner and travel companions. Let me tell you a little bit more about Mike, my wonderful boyfriend of ten years. Mike did all the photography for *Live Raw*, my first recipe book, and his photographs grace the pages of *Live Raw Around the World*. Mike carried all his camera equipment from country to country to capture thousands of scenery and food photos. He photographed immediately after I prepared and styled a dish so you could see how a meal looks when it's on the plate. He took photos of people, buildings, and everything he could so we could share some of the sights we experienced on our journey.

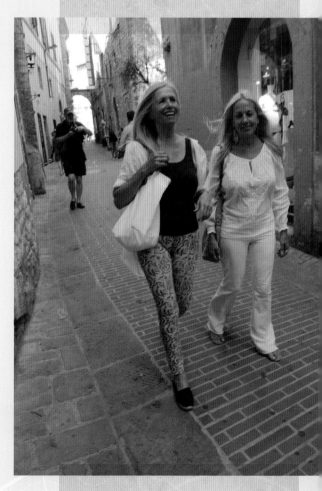

He is also the best recipe taster around. Poor guy, after he photographs all the food, he is duty-bound to taste-test everything. Luckily for me, he never complained—even after eating a third or fourth dessert. Without his help in all my life's latest endeavors, it just wouldn't be as much fun. I've traveled alone many times, but nothing compares to traveling with like-minded loved ones. Mike is more than just my right hand. He is a true partner in every sense of the word. I'm lucky and grateful to have him in my life.

We invited our close friends Michael Keller, a professional photographer, and his girlfriend, my dear friend Eileen Katzenstein, to join us in Italy and Greece. In the past, we've traveled to Michael's home on the East Cost as well as Eileen's charming homes in New York and Portugal. They both have extensive vegetable gardens, and we've enjoyed many raw meals together. Eileen loves to cook as much as I do, and both Michael and Eileen have daily green drinks. We share many common ideas about food and life. The four of us travel very well together, and we all had such a great, fun time on this journey.

I was excited when one of my daughters, Lisa, said she was able to join us on the India portion of our trip. Lisa and I had traveled abroad together before and always have an amazing time. She is a wonderful cook, as are all my children, and although she eats cooked food as part of a mostly plant-based diet, she includes raw foods and green drinks daily. She buys only organic, shops weekly at her local farmers market, and works in her community garden space, where she grows a variety of vegetables and herbs. Lisa is a superfoodie and loves to talk about food as much as I do. Once she started making raw zucchini pasta from her garden for friends, she turned a new group of people on to raw foods.

travel gift

Those of you who can't travel right now, don't worry: *Live Raw Around the World* is my gift to you, written and offered with love.

I brought information home on video, along with copious notes. I wrote while traveling, when we stopped for a meal, on trains, on planes, and in cars. I even wrote in the dark when I first woke up every morning and just before falling off to sleep each night. Many times I woke in the night to write a recipe that came into my mind while in that sleepy state. I gathered information from many new friends we met along the way, spent months in my kitchen measuring and calculating, and when I thought I was finished, I wrote and calculated some more. When it was all finally complete, I hoped it would become a gift that keeps on giving!

home delivery

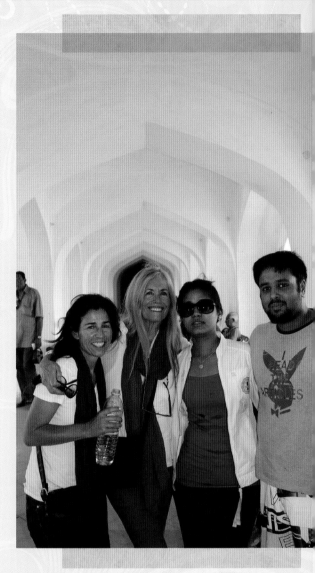

The world is full of many different cultures, and each has its own fascinating variety of flavors. We can't travel the world whenever or wherever we like, but that shouldn't stop us from enjoying international cuisine.

If you yearn for some travel but can't pick up and go right now, I'd like to minimize your longings. You won't need to pack a suitcase, grab a passport, or fasten your seat belt because the world will be transported to your door. In fact, I'm going to bring the world right into your kitchen.

I've chosen seven countries to broaden your culinary taste experience: Spain, France, Germany, Italy, Greece, India, and Thailand.

I've developed recipes incorporating fresh ingredients, spices, and herbs that are typical of each country. Step-by-step instructions will make it easy to create recipes from breakfast to dessert. Wherever you may live in the world, this book will enable you to buy locally and eat globally.

Live Raw Around the World will hopefully be your "go to" recipe book for exotic taste and international adventure. Treat yourself, family, and friends to healthy delicious global cuisine without leaving the comfort of your own home.

If you are lucky enough to travel and explore, anticipation will be around every corner. But alas, travel always comes to an end, and memories and photos are the precious commodities we have left to remember our trips.

Now you will have the luxury to recreate those lingering tastes and flavors with *Live Raw Around the World*. When you prepare some of the recipes, you will absorb the essence and aroma of each country.

lay of the land

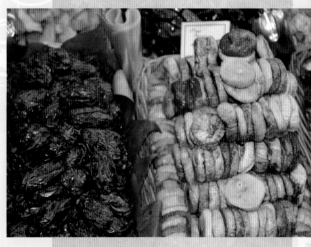

You can enjoy recipes by country, organized by breakfast, lunch, dinner, desserts, and drinks. Mixing and matching will make it easy to prepare complete courses with complementary flavors. Recipes ranging from raw versions of Spanish Pizza, Minestrone Soup, Portobello Steak au Poivre, Italian Spiced Stuffed Red Peppers, Spanish Vegetable Paella, Indian Curries, Pad Thai Noodles, Greek Wild Rice Stuffed Tomatoes, Tiramisu, Panna Cotta, and Spiced Chocolate Bark might just become favorites.

For those with limited local shopping options, most ingredients can be purchased online, including spices and herbs. (see p. 48) You will learn how to mix your own spices together to create new exotic tastes, making it possible for anyone to prepare these recipes wherever you might live in the world. Dining on international foods will transport the imagination *and* the taste buds, awakening the memories of the pleasures derived from a satisfying vacation.

In addition to the collection of recipes, you'll find highlights and stories from our traveling experiences. As you navigate through your own real-life journey, whether you are in your twenties, thirties, forties, fifties, sixties, or beyond, you will learn how you can improve your life in each moment. You will find information on longevity around the world and how it's possible to live a long, happy, healthy life wherever you may live. We'll explore processed foods and learn why these foods are so unhealthy for us and how chemicals, coloring, and additives in our food affect our overall health and well-being.

Health is at the heart of all the recipes, but so are taste and beauty. Setting the mood for each country's chapter, you'll find travel photographs, including farmers market stalls, local fresh vegetables, fruits, olives, spices, herbs, nuts, and scenery to inspire your senses.

Preparing raw food stimulates creativity, and the finished product can be a work of art. Food is part of our senses, including sight, taste, smell, touch, and feelings. If a meal is artfully arranged, it becomes an object of beauty and in turn excites the taste buds. The aroma of herbs and spices can make our mouths salivate. There is food we pick up and eat with our hands, and in many countries around the world it is the main way food is consumed. Taking a bite from a fresh, juicy, succulent mango or a slice of ice-cold watermelon reminds us of summer. Having a warm soup or cup of tea is soothing in winter. Food provides delight and satisfaction whether you're preparing it or consuming it.

It is much easier to stay on a healthy eating path without boredom if we know how to prepare a variety of raw foods. Keeping your refrigerator full of the right foods just makes it so much easier. There are times when we want a simple meal and other times we need something more complex. Knowing how to prepare a variety of foods will provide you with complete satisfaction on your path to ultimate health.

If you are looking to improve your diet, already love raw food, or are gluten sensitive, you will no doubt enjoy every recipe in this book from start to finish. If you are watching your weight or trying to heal yourself from ailments and disease, you will find many recipes that will help you achieve your goals. If you are new to some of the herbs and spices, I think you will find an exciting new taste experience. If you already love ethnic foods and have enjoyed eating them cooked, you will be happy to find a raw food version of some of your favorites. Whatever your interests, I'm happy you've joined me on this trip.

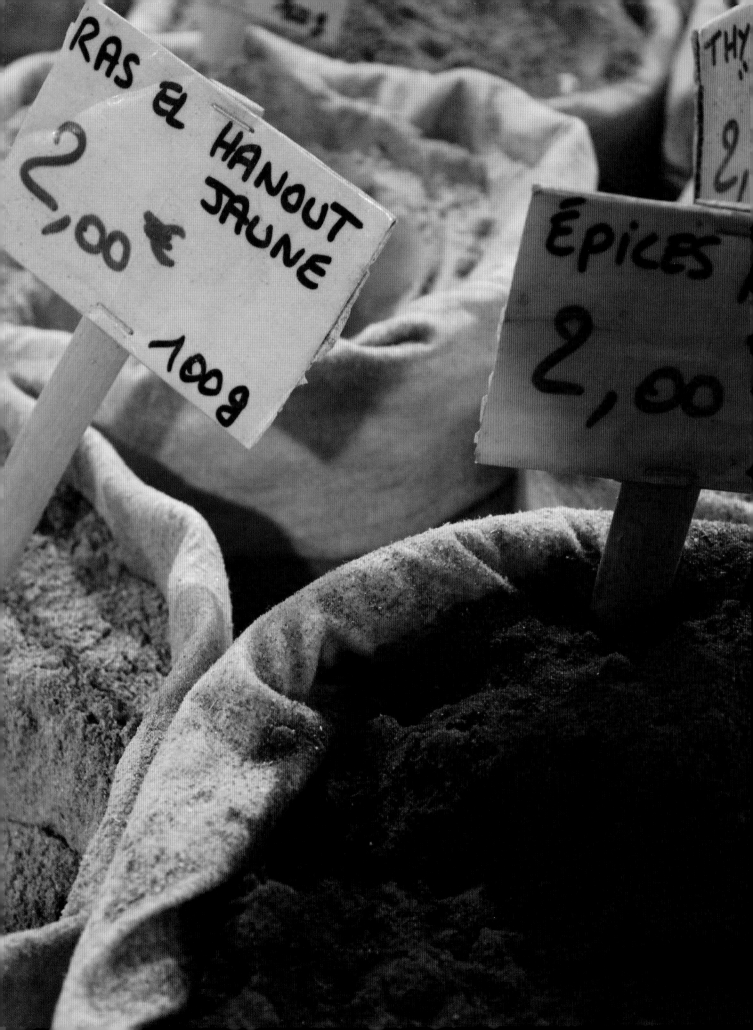

CHAPTER 2

··

CULTURES AND

FOOD

··

a world without borders

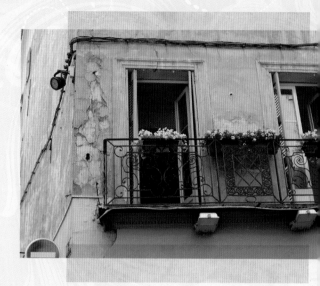

So many variations of the same dishes have traveled from country to country forgetting their origins. The world has become a gastronomic melting pot. There is a significant amount of adaptations of pizza in many countries, with each one having its own distinctive spices making it unique to its own heritage.

Although you will find versions of the same foods in many countries, each country continues to take pride in its own local cuisine, and no one could convince the locals that their classic ingredients are not the best in the world. The French, for instance, are very proud of their crepes. The Spaniards take satisfaction in paella, a rice dish, and the Germans love sauerkraut and sausages of any kind.

But it's not just about the food itself. For instance, Italians like to leisurely eat and drink with friends and family. They live *la dolce vita*, meaning "the sweet life," full of pleasure and indulgence. Food certainly plays a large part in this concept, but it's the enjoyment of life in general that they seek.

Italians are not the only ones. We found people all over the world who feel the same way. The Spaniards love to eat in restaurants and go from bar to bar eating tapas (small plates of food) while enjoying a drink and the company of friends late into the night. Indians are very family-oriented and prepare most meals at home. There is so much we can learn from each culture by keeping an open mind and heart.

language of food

Food is the mother of all language, a language we all understand regardless of culture. Fruits and vegetables are similar wherever you travel but expressed differently when prepared. Even in Italy or India, where locals use the same ingredients throughout the country, the cuisine is prepared differently from one region to another.

Food has many stories to tell—stories of origin, family, and history—and raw food has its own stories to tell as humans started out eating only raw food until fire was mastered. In ancient Greece, there was a religious school where the disciples were required to be vegetarians. Hippocrates, the father of medicine, said, "Let food be your medicine." Hippocrates was believed to be primarily a raw vegan. The famous fifteenth-century Italian painter Leonardo da Vinci was known to consume only a raw plant product-based diet, and it is said he lived mainly on a fruitarian diet.

> "Vitality and beauty are gifts of nature for those who live by her laws."
>
> ~ Leonardo da Vinci

Raw food recipes use many of the same basic ingredients as cooked foods, but we need to prepare them differently. Cooked rice can be long grain or short, whereas a raw food chef will sprout wild rice, buckwheat, or oat groats and make rice from parsnip, cauliflower, or jicama. Non-raw cooks prepare their beans in many different ways depending on where they live in the world. Some boil, some fry, and others refry them. Since raw foodists do eat most beans, a raw cook might sprout lentils, peas, chickpeas, or mung beans for a similar taste as cooked beans.

Sprouts are added to soups, chili, burgers, and salads. Whether cooked or raw, a variety of herbs and spices are ultimately important to achieve the flavor and essence of each country's cuisine.

Regardless of how a meal is prepared in any culture, food brings people together. A chef in any country can talk for hours about food, including what farm the food was purchased from or different ways to slice or dice a vegetable or the colors and arrangement of food on a plate. We can spend hours talking about garnishes, sauces, and salt. We even discuss food while we are sitting at a table enjoying a meal. If you share a love, passion, and commitment for good food, you will immediately have a friend in any country.

International food and wine festivals are popular events around the world, and depending on where we live, finding international restaurants in major cities and enjoying foods from other countries seems second nature.

Although some of these global restaurants may serve vegetarian food, finding raw vegan food in most can prove to be difficult or even impossible. The longing for international food is a challenge when adopting a raw food diet. In the last few years, I've made thousands of friends around the world on my social network pages that are now eating raw foods or who are trying to include more raw foods in their diets. We are all looking for a world of flavor, new methods of preparation of raw food, and exciting conversation with new friends at our dinner tables.

oh, the joy of farmers markets

In Tuscany, Italy, farmers markets are called *mercatali;* in Thailand they are called *talad*; in Spain they are simply known as street markets. Whatever their name, shopping at these colorful markets plays a key role in obtaining the freshest of foods in every country.

Farmers markets exist worldwide and are held in various neighborhoods, villages, and square on different days of the week. Many people shop daily, and others shop two or three times a week to purchase the freshest daily crops. We watched men and women carrying off their baskets or shopping bags filled with market finds, many stopping along the way for the ritual of meeting up and talking with friends.

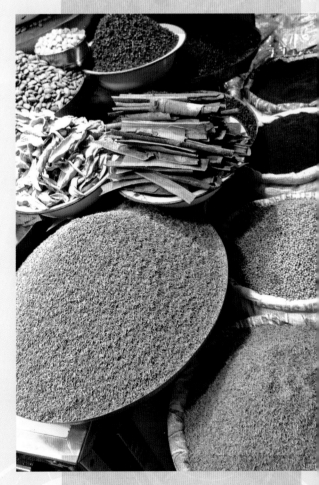

There is an excitement in discovering new varieties of local harvest fruits and vegetables. One can feel the enthusiasm and hustle and bustle of farmers setting up their stands, vendors shouting out the special of that day, and elderly women sorting their goods for sale while balancing on a small wooden box or tiny chair.

Vendors around the world take pride in what they grow and hope to sell their merchandise at the busy market that day. Some vendors have large stalls, and others have just a tiny, overloaded space, but large or small, they all have their own special style of display and selling.

There are stalls selling kitchenware, table covers, clothes, personal goods, local crafts, seeds, plants, flowers, olives, prepared foods, sundry items, and woven straw shopping baskets, a favorite of mine.

Shoppers can find heirloom varieties, certified organic produce, or conventional choices, and most markets are from drivable to walking distance from their homes.

Farmers pick produce when it is ripe and at its peak, which provides greater nutritional content and is far more flavorful.

Shopping at farmers markets is better for the environment because the local produce travels fewer miles to reach us, which definitely makes a lighter carbon footprint. It's also an excellent way to learn about an area's culture. People are friendly and open to share recipes and their way of life. When organic farmers sell wholesale to supermarkets, their profits are often quite small. Selling directly to the consumer helps smaller organic farmers stay in business and also helps preserve our natural resources. Farmers and vendors we met on our travels appreciated their hard-earned money going directly in their pockets and not to middlemen.

Farmers around the world love direct communication with their customers and feel rewarded when they see the same faces come back week after week. It's my pleasure to support organic farmers because their hard work brings us clean food to preserve our health while promoting the health of the soil.

Farm to table is the way I prefer my food, and I'm obviously not the only one. In the United States alone, farmers markets have grown from 1,755 in 1994 to 7,864 in 2012, with new markets opening rapidly every year.

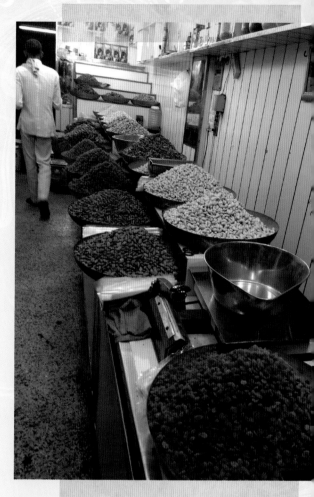

In most countries around the world and before modernization and supermarkets, street markets were the main source of buying produce. On this trip, I noticed more grocery stores opened in countries that had very few on my previous visits. Supermarkets sell packaged goods and produce that are being shipped in from all around the world. Although many locals still shop at the farmers markets, supermarkets are gaining in popularity. Just like in the United States, humans everywhere love convenience.

If you're not already shopping at farmers markets, you are missing out on a great experience as well as delicious fresh produce.

travel

(Ad-ven-ture) n. involvement in bold undertakings

It is easy to get stuck in the routines of daily life, dietary choices, and the safety and comforts of repetitive patterns, but once you step outside of your comfort zone and explore new places and experiences, I think you will agree that life is an amazing adventure to be lived to its fullest.

Try something new! Venture out! Explore! Be daring! Have courage! That's what life is all about. That's what travel is all about, and that is what food is all about. Enjoying raw international food and learning about people around the world allows us to feel connected to the world and the planet in a new and unique way. It makes it hard not to recognize our similarities to other women or men in other countries.

People everywhere want peace, happiness, and the best for their children and loved ones. We all laugh and cry. We all feel stress and joy. We are alike in so many ways. Building a happy, healthy environment is as important to others as it is to us. The love for good food is universal, especially when a meal is shared with others.

"The journey of a thousand miles begins with a single step."

~ Lao Tzu

Hollywood, California, is only a few hours from the Tijuana, Mexico, border. When I was young, my parents took us to Tijuana many times; in fact, it was the only place we ever traveled to. We would stay in San Diego overnight and then cross the border during the day. It was always fun and exciting to see local crafts and learn how other people lived in another country. Being from a lower-middle-class family and seeing others with much less than we had made me grateful for what I had. Mom always packed food for our trip, as Dad never let us eat in Mexico. My father and mother had no idea that I was eating Mexican food while still in grammar school. After school, most days I would walk to the Girls Club and spend time there before going home. Once or twice a week, there was a Mexican man who parked a small food cart in front of the club. I had seen these forbidden carts before, as they were the same ones my parents would never let me eat from on our trips to Tijuana. I would save my lunch money so I could buy a tamale from the cart's hot steamer. The gentleman would open the lid and pull out the hot tamale with tongs. He put the tamale in a cardboard dish, opened up the cornhusks, and filled the top of the tamale with chili and cheese. I would sit on the curb and enjoy every slightly spicy morsel. On the way home, I chewed gum to disguise my breath and hide my secret pleasure. My sister Arlene was my accomplice on many occasions, and our parents never found out our little secret.

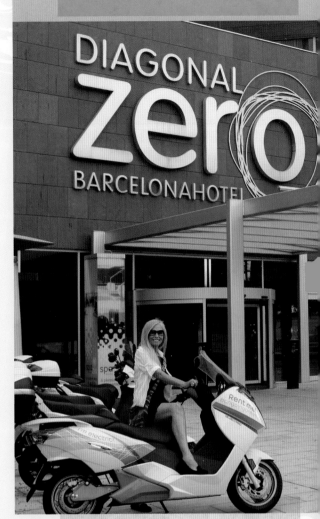

Tijuana was the extent of my travel until my early thirties, when I traveled with my boss, Valerie Harper, as she was making an appearance in London. We traveled from there to Italy for a vacation with some of her family members and her manager. While in England, on occasion it was my job to handle the money and figure out how to pay our taxi drivers in British pounds. It was so confusing that I just held out the money in my hands and let them take the appropriate amount. I did that several times before gaining some understanding of the pound.

Italy is where I fell deeply in love, not only with the country but also with travel in general. Once the travel bug bites, you're infected for life. When I got the first stamp on my passport, life was never the same again. In Italy I felt awestruck looking at the ancient buildings, ruins, massive marble statues, sidewalk cafes, fountains, people, and ambience in general. I felt so alive—a new world had opened up for me.

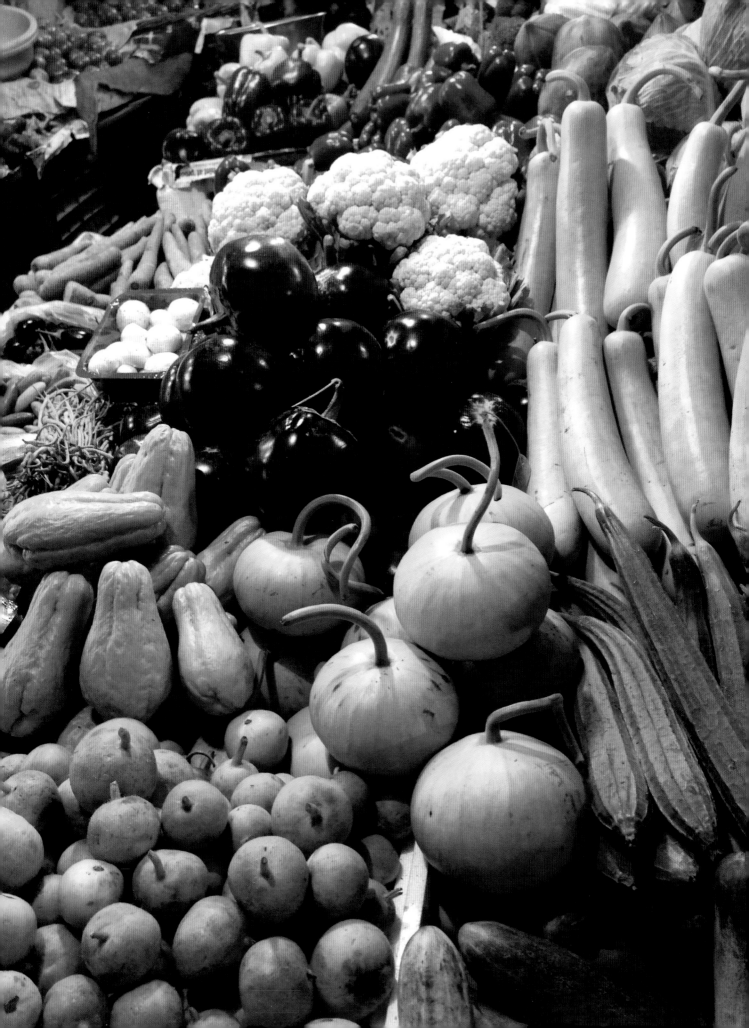

CHAPTER 3

·····················

ABOUT RAW

FOOD

·····················

protein guide

Let's just get right to it: protein. This is the first question everyone I meet asks: "How do you get your protein?" Meat is not the only source of protein, however. In fact, it's far from the best source. Greens are full of protein. Broccoli contains 45% protein compared to beef, which contains 25%. Spinach contains 49% compared to pork with only 27% and chicken with 23%. Kale contains 45% protein, parsley 34%, cauliflower 40%, cucumbers 24%, green pepper 22%, and mushrooms 37%. Tomatoes have 18% protein and eggs just 12%. So the protein myth that one needs meat is just that: a myth.

Sea vegetables and seaweed also have more protein than an egg. Sea vegetables contain more calcium per ounce than milk. If we eat a variety of plant foods, we are receiving adequate protein. The World Health Organization (WHO) claims we need only 5% of our daily calories to come from protein to be healthy. The U.S. Department of Agriculture (USDA) claims we need 6.5%, and the Centers for Disease Control recommend that 10–35% of our daily calories should come from protein. Confusing at it might seem, 20–50% of the calories

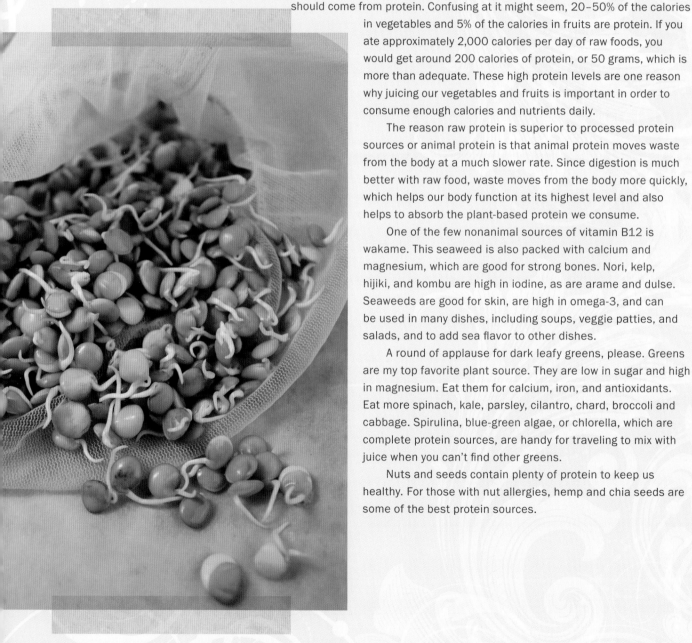

in vegetables and 5% of the calories in fruits are protein. If you ate approximately 2,000 calories per day of raw foods, you would get around 200 calories of protein, or 50 grams, which is more than adequate. These high protein levels are one reason why juicing our vegetables and fruits is important in order to consume enough calories and nutrients daily.

The reason raw protein is superior to processed protein sources or animal protein is that animal protein moves waste from the body at a much slower rate. Since digestion is much better with raw food, waste moves from the body more quickly, which helps our body function at its highest level and also helps to absorb the plant-based protein we consume.

One of the few nonanimal sources of vitamin B12 is wakame. This seaweed is also packed with calcium and magnesium, which are good for strong bones. Nori, kelp, hijiki, and kombu are high in iodine, as are arame and dulse. Seaweeds are good for skin, are high in omega-3, and can be used in many dishes, including soups, veggie patties, and salads, and to add sea flavor to other dishes.

A round of applause for dark leafy greens, please. Greens are my top favorite plant source. They are low in sugar and high in magnesium. Eat them for calcium, iron, and antioxidants. Eat more spinach, kale, parsley, cilantro, chard, broccoli and cabbage. Spirulina, blue-green algae, or chlorella, which are complete protein sources, are handy for traveling to mix with juice when you can't find other greens.

Nuts and seeds contain plenty of protein to keep us healthy. For those with nut allergies, hemp and chia seeds are some of the best protein sources.

about sprouting

One of the reasons for sprouting seeds and nuts is that it releases enzyme inhibitors, making it easier for our bodies to digest. Sprouting nuts is a little different from sprouting seeds, such as those of radishes, peas, lentils, chickpeas, alfalfa, and clover, to name a few, as these seeds grow a tail when sprouted and nuts don't. Nuts are considered sprouted when they are covered with pure water and soaked for four hours or overnight. Munch on a small amount of almonds, walnuts, and pecans for added protein. Nut butters can be made at home and are out of this world (see p. 55). Use cashews, almonds, or macadamia nuts to make cheeses and sauces. Snack on sunflower or pumpkin seeds, or make hemp milk and chia seed puddings.

Looking for some good protein sources all year around? You can't beat sprouted seeds and legumes. They can be added to salads, soups, or juices or eaten as a snack. Sprouts can be grown on your kitchen counter so you always have something fresh and alive, even in winter months. (For information on where to purchase seeds, see p. 209.)

raw food love

The way you choose to eat is always in flux when beginning the path to good health, as the old way of eating for emotional or social reasons continues to knock at your door. Listening to your body before and after eating is important. In this way you learn how food affects you. Processed foods are addictive and lead to cravings for more of the same. Many times after eating cooked food we feel full but not satisfied, so along comes another helping or a

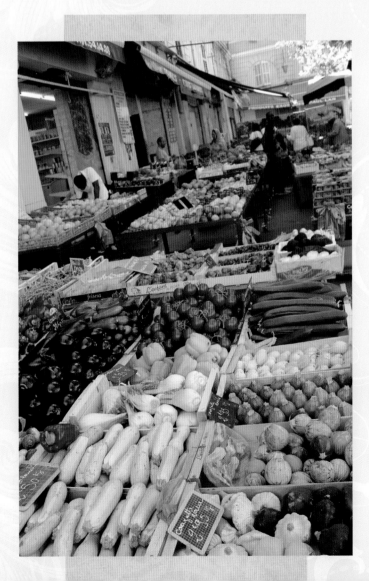

sugary dessert. Cooked food takes time to digest, and along with slow digestion, important nutrients that are lost in cooking are not giving your body the nourishment it needs, so we tend to overeat.

Raw food digests quickly because it retains enzymes. It sustains us longer after eating, and we get more nutrients than with cooked foods, so we feel satisfied more quickly. Pay attention after finishing a meal, and see if you notice the difference.

Balance is important. A balanced life is what you are aiming for. How you eat affects everything around you. I believe eating raw is the best you can do for yourself, but if family or social life makes it difficult, just do the best you can and keep moving in the right direction. Everyone's situation is different. For some, eating 75 to 90 percent raw works best. Eat as much raw food as you can, and don't forget to include your green drink or smoothie every day.

When food is cooked, the flavors and textures are brought out in a variety of ways, including steaming, sautéing, roasting, or baking. The human race has learned many techniques and methods over time to make food tasty. When it comes to raw food, using spices and herbs, dehydrating, and marinating are the main ways to make raw foods expand their natural flavors. It takes time to learn something new, but remember when you first learned to cook, it took years to perfect your cooking skills. Be patient, and you will soon be comfortable preparing delicious, healthful, raw food meals.

Many young men and women don't know how to cook because they grew up in a time when their mothers, who were once stay-at-home moms, became part of the workforce outside the home. A young girl once told me she didn't cook, but she knew how to heat. She said she bought prepared foods exclusively and learned how to warm them.

Learning how to prepare your own food at home can improve your health. If you don't spend some time preparing food at home, you will be subjected to eating restaurant or fast food that might not be healthy. Although it might taste good, powerful questions remain: What chemicals are you consuming? What cooking methods were used? How much salt or trans fat does it contain? And will it be good for your health in the long run, or will it eventually make you sick?

Some raw foodists consider dehydrated foods gourmet. My personal taste is to eat simply most days and include lots of salads. But without some of these little special dehydrated treats, I don't know if I would enjoy staying raw all the time. Crackers, breads, warm lasagna, sprouted wild rice, cookies, and kale chips are all made in a dehydrator. Granola, stuffed peppers, pizza crust, and so many other tasty dishes are all dehydrated. A dehydrator might just become one of your favorite kitchen tools.

Shopping, preparing, and sharing food is something I enjoy. Hanging out in the kitchen preparing food with family and friends might not be for everyone, and that is why fast food has become so popular. However, more recently, people are learning that fast foods are far from the ideal way to eat, and eating habits are starting to change around the world.

If you are new to raw food, it's always good to start slowly and learn to make some of your favorite cooked "go to" dishes into raw "go to" dishes. This way you will be less tempted to eat foods that are not good for you. A great way to start is by cutting out all processed foods (eat nothing in a box, bag, can, or pouch) and eating only fresh foods, as close to natural as possible. Just by taking this step, you will be well on your way to better health. The less processed food you eat, the healthier you will be.

starting a raw food lifestyle

It's not about being perfect or giving up delicious food; it's about a new limitless adventure in foods and optimum health. This lifestyle and way of eating is essentially preventative medicine. Here's how to get started:

1. Make friends with others who already eat raw food. There are many raw potluck groups around the country. Check the Internet for one in your community.
2. Become friends on Facebook and Twitter with other raw foodists, many of whom love to talk and share recipes and ideas.
3. Google raw food websites and blogs. There is always new, eye-opening information to read.

4. Write down any changes you see in yourself after eating a plant-based meal. Notice your energy level, your digestion, and whether or not you feel satisfied after eating.

5. Remind yourself why you decided to eat raw, vegan, or vegetarian. Now is a perfect time to give yourself a pat on the back!

6. Read labels on any packaged food in your cupboard. If you don't know how to pronounce some of the ingredients, then it's time to clean out your pantry of all processed foods. Give or throw them away so you are not tempted to eat them.

7. Buy a good high-speed blender like a Vitamix or Blendtec. If you can't afford a new one, Vitamix sells reconditioned ones. If you can't afford either of those options, buy a less expensive blender and start saving up for a good one. You might also find a juicer at a garage sale or on Craigslist. Both blender and juicer are important in a raw food diet.

8. Detoxify your body for 3–7 days, drink vegetable juice and smoothies, and eat salads. Add fruit to your vegetable juice for a sweeter taste. I recommend apples or berries. Cut out all oils and fats, including avocado while you are detoxifying. Use apple cider vinegar, lemon, or a little apple juice on salads, and add herbs or spices to your salad to punch up the taste. Don't go hungry. If you need more food, fix another juice or have another salad or piece of fruit. Detoxifying will help toxic waste and unwanted pounds leave your body.

9. A dehydrator can be very handy. If you can't afford an Excalibur or Weston, find an inexpensive one at a garage sale or on Craigslist. A dehydrator will provide variety in preparing foods. You can make breads, crackers, cookies, and warm foods. You can also make kale and corn chips and other healthful snack foods.

10. **Do not try to convince anyone else to eat raw food:** not your family, not your friends, and especially not your mate. Anyone not educated about raw food will say you will not get enough protein and that you need to eat meat. There is time for sharing down the line.

11. Do what's best for you right now, and focus on your own well-being.

12. Hang out with other like-minded people, who have similar views not only in the area of food but also regarding the quality of life.

13. When your change is obvious, people will start asking you questions, and then would be the better time to share your experience.

14. When you think friends are ready, a good casual way to introduce them to raw food is to serve them a raw dessert. Cheesecake, pie, chocolates, or cookies always go a long way in educating people about how delicious raw food can be.

15. Don't be hard on yourself if you go off track. Remember: Just keep moving in the right direction.

healthy steps for busy people

You've made a commitment to yourself, and you need to create new habits. Planning ahead saves time in the long run, and taking care of your health now saves your life in the long run.

1. Plan your menu weekly. If you know what you're going to eat and have all the ingredients readily available, you will save time both mentally and physically.

2. Shop once a week.

3. Arrive home and store your vegetables properly in your refrigerator. Do not wash anything. Wrap vegetables in paper towels, and place them in plastic bags or containers. Wash only when ready to use. Mark the bag or container so you can quickly find what you're looking for.

4. Once a week make breads, crackers, veggie patties, cookies, granola, and hummus, the things you can grab when you are on the go. These can be made in the evening, dehydrated overnight, and stored in a container or refrigerator.

5. Perfect a handful of meals, and once you have mastered their preparation, they will be easy and quick to duplicate.

6. Eat simply. Salads take no time at all to prepare. Zucchini pasta is a snap and can be warmed or eaten at room temperature and served with a variety of toppings. Once veggie patties are made, you can have a delicious sandwich in just minutes by putting one between lettuce or Savoy cabbage leaves and adding dressing, avocado, tomato, red onion, or sprouts to have a quick, satisfying meal.

7. Smoothies are always satisfying and quick. You can turn a green smoothie or juice into a delicious soup by adding spices and herbs. Make a warm soup with fresh tomatoes, soaked sun-dried tomatoes, spinach, onion, garlic, celery, and carrot. Add herbs, blend until smooth, pour on top of finely chopped vegetables, including sweet red pepper, celery, carrots, cilantro, sweet red onion, and avocado, and you have a beautiful, quick, satisfying meal in minutes.

raw food can change your life

Amazing things happen when you start a raw food lifestyle. Simplicity in eating fresh raw food can change your emotional outlook. You may discover you have a different purpose in life than you previously thought. You may find a new freedom along the way. You might even discover a new joy, peace, and happiness in your life.

Many men and women who begin eating a raw food diet feel so good, they decide to help others improve their health. Some make a decision to make raw food a health and a profession. There are many chefs, consultants, authors, speakers, and coaches who can help you achieve this goal. (To learn more about becoming a professional, see p. 210.)

Brand yourself and your message. What will be your specialty? What subject and experience can you teach others? What changed for you once you started eating raw food? Start a blog to share your experience. Learn to share your message in front of others. Join a local Toastmasters club (there are many meeting groups worldwide). At Toastmasters, you will learn how to hone your speaking and leadership skills in a no-pressure atmosphere. You can share your passion with others and learn to take your message out to the public. Many speakers make good incomes, travel the world, and educate others with their message.

Raw food can make you feel healthier than you have in your entire life. The changes you see in your internal and external body will give you a new lease on life. Look forward to a new opportunity for happiness. Taking care of your health gives you a better outlook on life. Your clear eyes and happy smile will be obvious to those around you.

"We are living in a world today where lemonade is made from artificial flavors and furniture polish is made from real lemons."

~ Alfred E. Newman

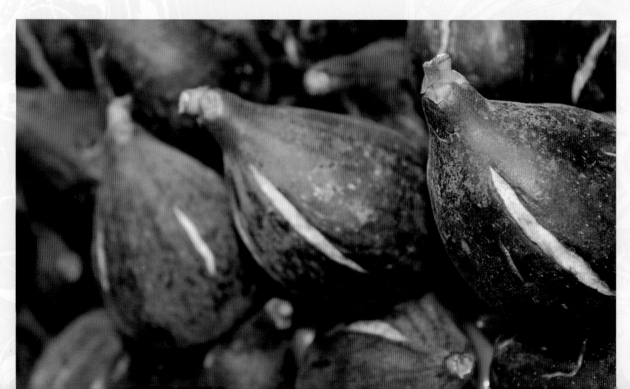

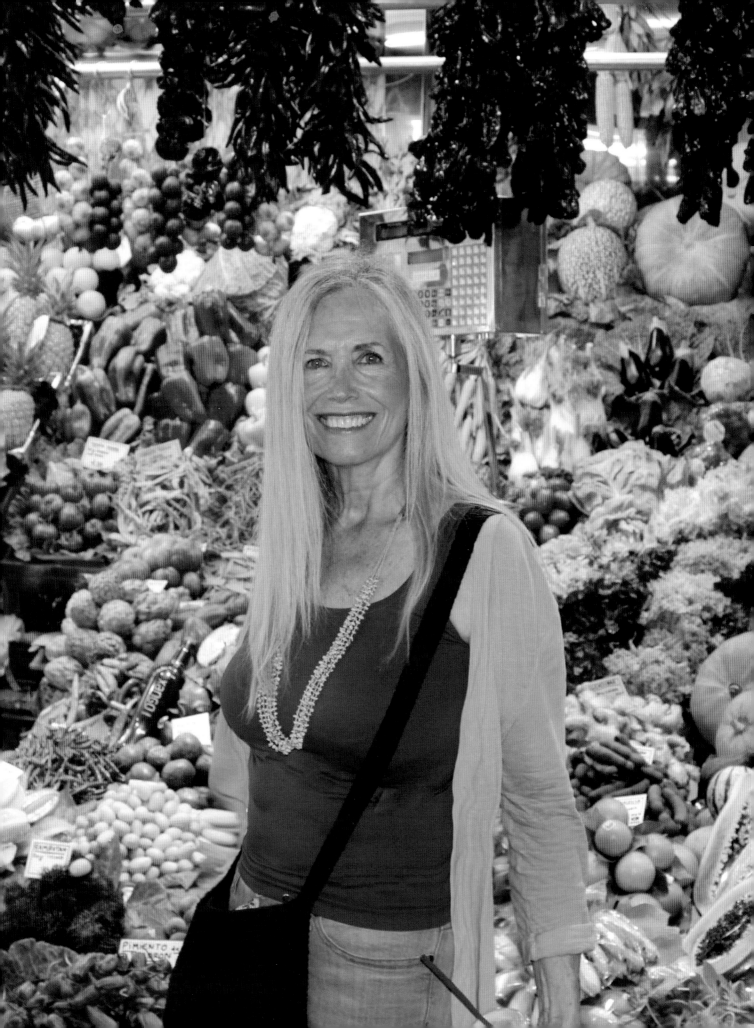

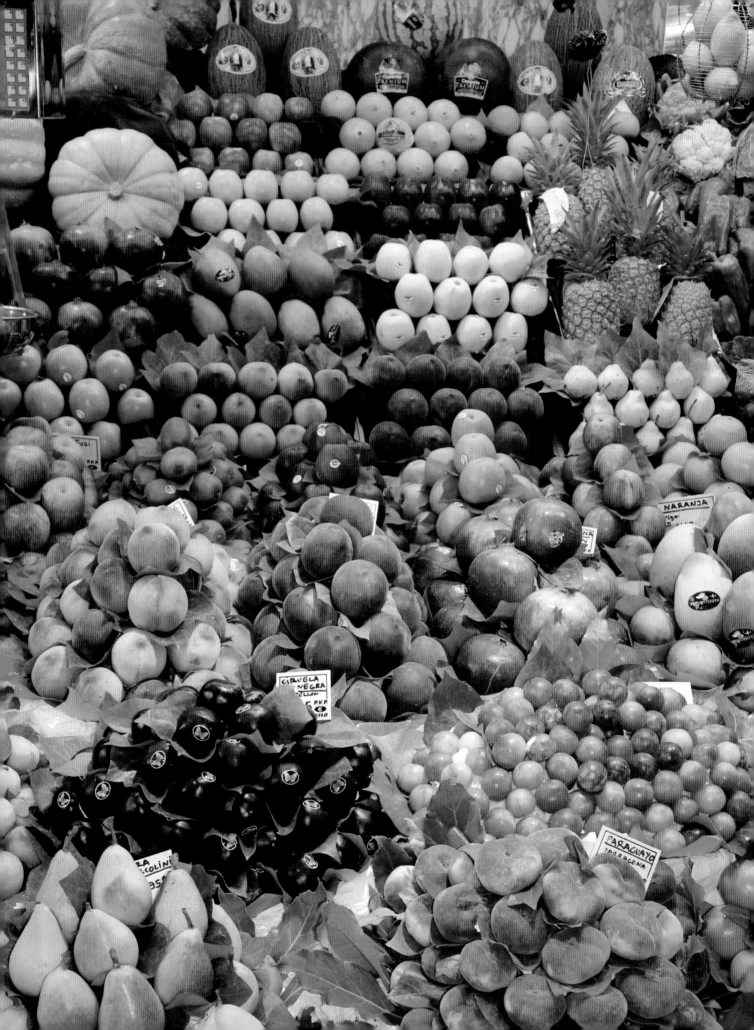

CHAPTER 4

· · · · · · · · · · · · · · · · · · · ·

LET'S TALK FOOD BEFORE

WE EAT

· · · · · · · · · · · · · · · · · · · ·

what we don't know can hurt us

Some of you might have heard the old saying, "What you don't know can't hurt you." I disagree with this statement, and I'm going explain why using three literary characters.

Character number one: I would like to introduce you to the antagonists . . . you know, like the Borg in *Star Trek*, the Joker in *Batman*, Darth Vader in *Star Wars*, Lex Luthor in *Superman*, the Wicked Witch of the West in *The Wizard of Oz*, or Cruella De Vil in *101 Dalmatians*. Of course, these are all movie antagonists, so we're not really afraid of them. What we might be afraid of, however, are the real-life antagonists, including attention-deficit/hyperactivity disorder (ADHD), arthritis, asthma, cancer, diabetes, depression, heart attack, high blood pressure, high cholesterol, memory loss, obesity, chronic fatigue, osteoporosis, Parkinson's, and strokes, to name just a few. If we're not personally trying to get rid of one or more antagonists, we probably know someone who is.

Character number two: The allies. The allies are the antagonists' best friends. They help keep the antagonists alive and make it possible for them to continue their evil deeds. If you notice, all antagonists have allies in films, and the same applies to real life. Meet a few real-life allies that fall into the category of processed foods: monosodium glutamate, dyes, high-fructose corn syrup, sodium, antibiotics, steroids, hormones, fortified vitamins, trans fats, refined grains, and solvents. There are over 6,000 chemicals and additives common in food today, and too many for me to mention here. These real-life allies are the reason for the antagonists' existence.

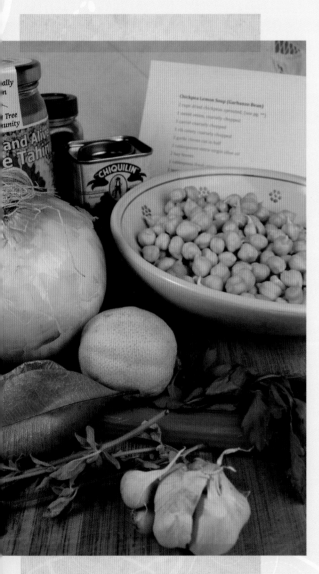

Where do these allies live? They exist in processed foods, which are quick and easy to prepare or eat right from the box or bag. Processed food is anything altered from its natural state. If it's bagged, boxed, or in a pouch or can, it's more than likely processed. Before putting anything in your shopping cart, read the label. Don't trust the advertising on the front of the package. Manufacturers will say anything to get you to buy their products, but with closer examination of the ingredient list, you will find that processed foods today are filled with chemicals, dyes, and fortified vitamins, which our bodies don't assimilate. A package may say blueberry cereal when, in fact, there are no blueberries in the box. Many carrot cake mixes are carrot-less, made with carrot-flavored pieces that are derived from corn syrup, chemicals, and artificial colors, including yellow dye #6 and red dye #40. Manufacturers use dyes in cereals and candy to make them more "fun" for kids.

Many color dyes have been linked to ADHD and behavioral problems in children. Dyes can also cause brain cell toxicity. Food companies use dyes because synthetic dyes are cheaper to use than real ingredients. The manufacturers of many fruit drinks let you think their drinks contain cherries and berries, when there are zero percent berries and cherries in the actual drink.

Since 1931, a highly toxic ingredient has been added to citrus-flavored soft drinks as a clouding agent and emulsifier. Manufacturers take bromine and mix it with vegetable oil and call it brominated vegetable oil or BVO. Most people have never heard of BVO because they never look at the ingredients in the products they consume. Even if they did, they would not know what BVO was unless they took the time to look it up. Take a look at a can or bottle of sports drinks, carbonated sodas, or soft drinks, and you will see BVO mentioned. BVO can also be found in some bakery goods and pastas. BVO is also used in printing papers, additives for gasoline, and agricultural fumigants. BVO can cause iodine deficiency and is a potential carcinogen. If you knew about this chemical, would you want to drink it or give it to your children?

More than 100 countries ban BVO. The Center for Science in the Public Interest and the Food and Drug Administration list BVO as an additive in the same category as aspartame and quinine. We are told there is a very small amount in our soft drink and we would have to consume a large amount for it to negatively affect us. Many people, however, have been diagnosed with problems caused by BVO buildup in their systems, such as confusion, headaches, memory loss, kidney disease, weight gain, heart problems, fatigue, and cancer.

Gathering ammunition for a talk I was giving, I came across a box of cereal I loved as a child. These days that particular company has thirteen different kinds of cereal on the shelves. One box showed a picture of a woman exercising, and the box claimed you'd lose weight, look better, and get healthier eating its cereal. When you read the ingredients, however, you get a different picture. The box claims the cereal has several different grains. It never mentions that processing the grains removed much of the vitamins and minerals. Another list appears below the ingredients claiming the addition of fortified vitamins and minerals. Fortified vitamins are synthetically engineered. Research shows that our bodies don't recognize or absorb synthetic vitamins and they get stored in our body as fat. Many times manufacturers add ingredients as a tease to make us think their product is healthier than their competition, but in fact there may be too much sugar, salt, or fats for it to be considered healthy. Don't be fooled by advertising on processed food packaging. The more hype, the more you should question the ingredients.

Another of my supermarket finds was a can of soup targeted at children. Manufacturers may put photos of cartoon characters on their labels. You might recognize the cartoon character, but the unrecognizable names in the ingredients read like a list of scientific chemicals, not something you would want to feed your child. Often the list includes different names for monosodium glutamate (MSG). It's illegal to give your children cigarettes and alcohol, but it's not illegal to put MSG in their food? MSG is in 80% of our processed food. It might be called by one of the forty names used to disguise MSG, including modified food starch, tapioca starch, hydrolyzed vegetable protein (HVP), yeast extract, vegetable protein extract, and artificial flavorings, just to name a few. MSG is a flavor enhancer that can cause brain damage, retinal degeneration, behavior disorders, learning disabilities, obesity, and much more.

If you read labels, be sure to look at the portion size. For example, in the freezer department you can find a chicken potpie with 580 calories and 880 grams of sodium. A closer look at the label will reveal that the chicken pie was meant for two servings. If you consume the whole pie yourself, and that's what usually happens, you've consumed 1,100 calories and 1,700 grams of sodium—too much if you are concerned about your health.

Many toxic ingredients may not be recognizable on the label. The names of obvious chemicals have been changed to protect the manufacturers, not us, the consumers. The rule is: Do not eat any processed food unless you know what all the ingredients are.

Do you make popcorn in your microwave? A study published recently in the *Journal of the American Medical Association* found that nonstick chemicals in popcorn bags, and in many pots, baking sheets and pans, might damage the immune system. Microwaveable popcorn bags contain a chemical that prevents sticking and grease leakage. This chemical can lead to high cholesterol, sperm damage, infertility, and (ADHD). When our immune system is compromised, it can open the doors to many other health problems.

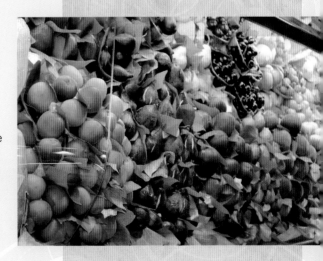

As you can see by now, we must take our health into our own hands and not trust what food manufacturers tell us. Processed food is making us fat and sick. Manufacturers are not concerned with our health; they are only concerned with sales. Read ingredients before you put any item into your shopping cart. If you can't pronounce the ingredients or you don't know what they are, put it back on the shelf until you can do some research.

Have you ever wondered about the expiration date on processed foods or why food last for years? Manufacturers use chemicals that prolong a product's shelf life, but they may have the opposite effect on our life.

To the Hindu, the cow represents all other creatures. Hindus believe that all living creatures are sacred, including mammals, fishes, and birds.

Did you know that certain hormones, antibiotics, and steroids we use in America for cattle are banned in the European Union? Australia, Canada, and Japan are just a few of the countries banning these hormones. The European Union has banned the import of meat from animals given these hormones.

Animals are not considered anything but a product to factory farmers. The latter seem to have forgotten that animals are living creatures. Many farmers are solely concerned with making their operation more profitable. Today, cows produce 40 percent more milk than they did years ago. Products such as recombinant bovine growth hormone (rBGH) and recombinant bovine somatotropin (rBST), one of the products manufactured by the Monsanto Company, are given subcutaneously in the tail, head, or behind the shoulder every fourteen days starting the ninth week of lactation to increase milk production. The safety of these drugs is questionable for both humans and animals. Synthetic hormones are known to increase an infection of the udder, which causes blood and pus to secrete into the milk, which leads to the need for more antibiotics. These drugs in humans can lead to prostate, breast, and colon cancers.

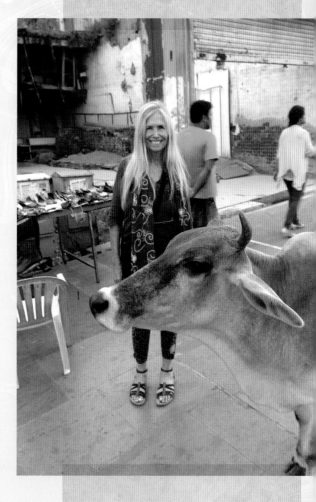

Antibiotics are mixed with the animals' feed or water as a preventive measure against disease. They also help cattle grow more quickly so they reach their desired slaughter weight faster. Even if only one cow is ill, the entire herd will receive medication to prevent any possible spread of disease. If you still consume milk, it must be organic and labeled rBST- and rBGH-free, or you are consuming exactly what the cow was given. Cheese is produced from the milk of cows that have been given antibiotics, hormones, and steroids. There is little doubt that we consume these drugs when we consume cheese.

I hope you've learned something more about processed foods and what they are doing to our health. I also hope you are inspired to clean out your cupboards of any foods that do not support a healthy lifestyle.

Character number three: It's time to introduce you to the heroes. Heroes are always great benefactors of humankind. A hero expands people's sense of what is possible for human beings. In movies, we all love when the heroes appear: James Bond, Indiana Jones, Robin Hood, Joan of Arc, Superman, and Luke Skywalker, to name a few. But the heroes I'm going to introduce to you are our real-life heroes. You already know them by name: apples, carrots, dark leafy greens, cucumbers, zucchini, strawberries, bananas, celery, sweet peppers, cabbage, broccoli, pineapples, and there are many more. No label to read and no expiration date necessary. With all their nutrients, vitamins, and minerals, they drive the antagonists away. The antagonists cannot survive where there are heroes. You and I are the allies to the heroes in a mutually beneficial arrangement, and all we have to do is make the choice for the betterment of our health by choosing the heroes. The more heroes we consume in their natural state, the greater chance we have of defeating the antagonists.

Fresh vegetables can play many roles. They can morph into many delicious meals. A zucchini, for example, can be baked, broiled, grilled, chopped into salads, used for breads, and made into raw pasta noodles for spaghetti and lasagna. Vegetables and fruits are beautiful to look at with their array of colors and shapes. They are full of all the nutrients that our bodies need to stay healthy. They are our real-life allies, the good guys. Eat them!

Please try to buy food labeled 100% organic. Genetically modified organisms (GMOs) do not have to be labeled in the United States, although they are required to be labeled in Europe. The most common GMO products are alfalfa, soybeans, corn, canola, sugar beets, papaya (especially from Hawaii), cotton, rice, dairy, aspartame, zucchini, and yellow summer squash, just to name a few. You can trust organic certifications including OAI, Oregon Tilth, and CCOF. However, USDA-certified organic standards might not be considered 100% organic and could still contain some GMO. The following sites can help you learn more and stay informed about GMOs: www.organicconsumers.org

www.nongmoproject.org/learn-more

There are many informative and interesting films on the subject of the foods we consume, including *Forks Over Knives; Food Matters; Food Inc.; Earthlings; Fast Food Nation; Fresh; The Future of Food; A Delicate Balance; Genetic Roulette; The World According to Monsanto; Bad Seed: The Truth About Our Food; Seeds of Freedom; Food Fight; Killer at Large; The Real Dirt on Farmer John; Patent for a Pig; The Beautiful Truth; Fat, Sick, and Nearly Dead; Dirt! The Movie;* and *King Corn.*

"It's bizarre that the produce manager is more important to my children's health than the pediatrician."

~ Meryl Streep

steps for living a long, healthy, and happy life

"Age is an issue of mind over matter. If you don't mind, it doesn't matter."

~ Mark Twain

longevity

Ideas for staying young:

1. Don't complain about your health.
2. Keep learning.
3. Invent new things to do daily.
4. Be upbeat; have a positive outlook on life.
5. Don't stress about things you can't change and focus on what you can.
6. Be satisfied and grateful for what you have, and don't dwell on what you don't have.
7. Be social with others; friends and family are important.
8. Maintain healthy habits.
9. Take care of your teeth.
10. Be active.
11. Put a smile on your face.
12. Be positive about your life.

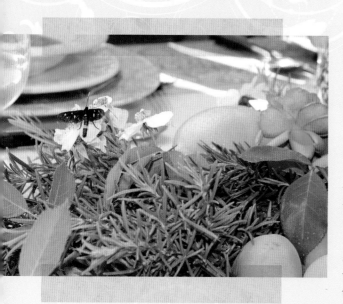

> "The secret to staying young is to live honestly, eat slowly, and lie about your age"
>
> ~ Lucille Ball

My sister Arlene and I are guardians for our oldest sister Sydell, who was never married or had children. Sydell was a resident in a senior assisted-living home in Northern California, and we recently moved her nearer us in Southern California to keep a closer eye on her. It was such a revelation going from one assisted-living residence to another to find her a home where we thought she would be happy.

Watching older people go through the motion of their daily lives, I wondered if they would have needed assisted living if they had taken better care of their health. While they are living long lives, could the quality be better? Most men and women in these facilities use walkers or are in wheelchairs. Some walk on their own, but they do not look like other seniors I know who are the same age but eat right and exercise. Many in these homes even look sedated. It's not exactly that assisted living is a bad thing; my sister lives in a nice home, for example. But it's still not what I see or want for my future. My sister enjoys assisted living. Her room is made up daily, and she has food 24/7 if she wants. She never liked to cook, so she is quite content that all her meals are prepared for her. She has constant company and planned activities. All her needs are looked after, and she feels safe not living alone.

There are 40 million people age sixty-five plus in the United States. It's predicted that by 2030, there will be more than 72 million seniors. There is no doubt we are living longer, but are we living healthier? The U.S. Center for Medicare and Medicaid Services estimates that about 9 million men and women over the age of sixty-five need long-term care. By 2020, that number is expected to rise to 12 million. A study by the U.S. Department of Health and Human Services says that four out of every ten people who reach age sixty-five will enter a nursing home at some point in their lives. These are alarming numbers and another reason to start taking better care of our health.

If you don't want to be one of those statistics, there are alternatives. Studies have been done on longevity, and men and women around the world who live the longest have many similarities.

When I was in my twenties and thirties, I thought that if I lived to be in my seventies that would be fantastic. But the older I get, the more years I want to live. Some time ago, I started to wonder if it was possible for me to live a long life. Some of my family members lived long, but they all had many age-related diseases. Researchers claim that less than 25 percent of how long and healthy the average person lives is dictated by genes. This means it's up to each individual to make choices that promote health and well-being. By making some simple changes, we can improve our lifestyle, look and feel better, and add years to our life expectancy.

diet

So how can we live longer? Does diet help? Is keeping healthy based on physical activity? Does our mind play a part in how long we live? There are several things that can help us live longer and healthier. Diet is at the top of the list. Research shows that the longest living people in the world eat primarily a plant-based diet. The ones who live the longest and also consume meat, fish, or tofu eat only small amounts of those, and usually only once or twice a week. A raw plant-based diet can help keep our digestive system healthy and functioning properly. A raw plant-based diet is proven to slow the effects of aging and provide enhanced energy.

When we take a look at schools, hospitals, and senior centers, we wonder how the food they serve in institutions can be healthy. In 2005, a British man named Jamie Oliver initiated a campaign called "Feed Me Better" in order to move British schoolchildren towards eating healthful foods and cutting out junk food. In 2010, he traveled to America to create the television series *Jamie Oliver's Food Revolution*, for which he went to Huntington, West Virginia, and then to Los Angeles to change the way Americans eat and address their dependence on fast food. Oliver brought attention around the world to the food served in our school lunch program. He noticed childhood obesity was an epidemic on the rise and that many meals children were fed at home were either packaged or fast food. Being a father himself, he felt that children should at least get one healthful meal a day and that school lunches were far from nutritious. Oliver believed that behavior and concentration in the classroom after lunch could be improved with proper healthful lunches. He wanted schools to start serving food that was fresh, high in nutrition, and not sugar-laden. Oliver also felt that teaching children about fresh foods at an early age would help them make better food choices throughout their lives and avoid obesity, diabetes, and vitamin deficiencies. With much

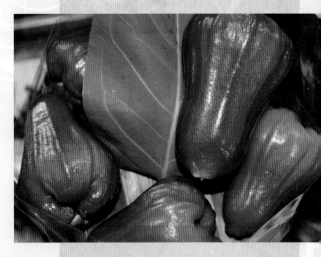

work and tenacity, he has accomplished numerous changes in school lunches that are being put into practice at a steady rate. He continues to be an activist, improving school lunch programs around the world. He is not a vegetarian or vegan, but I love this guy for all he does for children and parents who aren't aware of the importance of making better food choices.

If you've ever had a stay or visited a friend or family member in a hospital, then you will be familiar with this next topic: hospital food. I can only say it is quite shocking. Hospitals may have the latest technology, but the food is left back in the dark ages. Eggs, cheese, milk, bacon or sausage, instant oatmeal, nondairy creamer, and processed orange juice are on the trays of a hospital breakfast. Lunches and dinners are no improvement, with breaded fish and cream sauce, corn, a soft white-flour roll, cookies, and a tiny salad, which are considered a nutritious meal by hospitals. Don't forget the Jell-O and popsicles laden with sugar given to patients just out of surgery. I suppose the hospitals want to make sure the patient returns for another stay. My point is to take care of yourself, spend money on organic food when possible, stay away from processed foods, and eat fresh vegetables and fruit daily. In the long run, you will save money on doctor bills and avoid hospital stays (and hospital food!)

exercise

Almost everyone will agree that exercise is important, but how much is necessary to keep healthy and fit? Many people spend hours at the gym or run many miles on a daily basis. There has always been conflicting information about how much exercise is necessary. Some say twenty minutes a day will provide the same benefits as someone who works out for many hours every day. Others say just being active is enough. When it comes down to it, it all depends on your personal fitness goals. As adults, brisk walking, gardening, dancing, jogging, aerobics at least two and a half hours weekly can keep us in good shape. If that small amount of time doesn't fit into your schedule, the important key is that some exercise is better than none. If you can't work out every day, don't let that stop you from doing something. When shopping at the mall or supermarket, park far from the entrance so you can do some walking. Try taking the stairs instead of the elevator whenever possible. Take a walk break during lunchtime.

Studies published in *The Journal of Physiology* found that short periods of high-interval training were just as effective as long durations of endurance training. High-interval training may help improve metabolic health and could reduce the risk of chronic diseases, but it is not for everyone. Yoga, Pilates, qigong, and walking suit many people better. The idea is to find what works best for you and do it daily. If you can't find one hour to improve and maintain your health, you need to reschedule your calendar and book yourself in for an appointment. Without exercise, you might not enjoy your later years in good physical health. Find ways to make daily chores a little inconvenient so you use your body more. Remember, muscles need to be used or they wither, and the older you get, the faster you lose muscle tone if you are not exercising.

socializing

We are social creatures, and it's important for our lives to be filled with meaningful relationships. Hopefully those relationships are not diminished with age but grow even deeper. My mother outlived four of her children. I can hardly imagine what that felt like for her. She was not a religious woman, but she said a quiet prayer and lit candles for her deceased parents and children every Friday night for as long as I can remember. My mother held a happy, positive outlook on life and passed at ninety-five. She was a beautiful, loving, kind woman.

Much can happen as we age regarding loss of friends and loved ones. Research claims that one in three people in their sixties are chronically lonely, and a host of ills can occur—from high blood pressure to Alzheimer's—from loneliness. Creating and maintaining social relationships is very important as we age. It's also very important that older people have family and friends they can rely on, someone who can help keep their finances organized, make sure they have the right medication, and someone who just has their back in general. Keeping up with current events, volunteering, being involved in our community, and mentoring can keep us young.

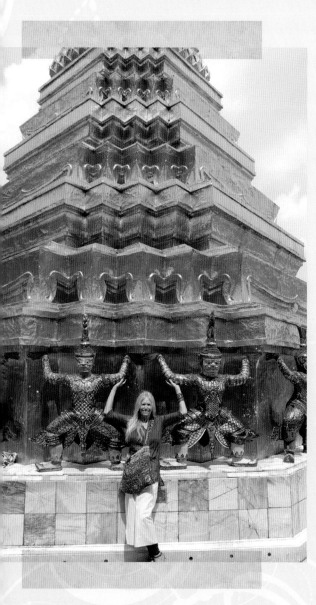

late bloomers

Age is not an issue. One of Grandma Moses' paintings sold for $1.2 million in 2006, and she only took up art at the age of seventy-five. Similarly, I run a business, lecture around the world, and just had my third book published. Other late bloomers include Colonel Sanders, founder of Kentucky Fried Chicken, who was sixty-five when he started his business, and went on to become a multimillionaire (I know, fried chicken?). You might remember Clara Peller, who was a manicurist before being hired as an actress at age eighty-one for the iconic Wendy's commercial with the line, "Where's the beef?" The actor Tony Randall fathered his first child with his fifty-year-younger wife at age seventy-five. Two years later he fathered his second child. Julia Child, not such a late bloomer by today's standards, published her first book at forty-nine, and her television program *The French Chef* first aired when she was fifty-one. My last, but not least, example is Maya Angelou, who was in her sixties when her poetry and books became popular.

"Having passion and an interest in life can keep us young."
~ Mimi Kirk

stereotyping and attitude

Aging gets a bad rap. Why is it that all older people are placed into a category called "the elderly"? We are labeled and not always in a positive way. We were all different from one another in our early years, so why would those traits disappear because we are older? I admit, some of my ideas have changed. I dropped much of the worry I had in my younger years concerning supporting my family, honing my parenting skills, and improving my relationships, but I'm still the same person. I still feel very young and optimistic, and my health is excellent. If I'm lucky, I might have thirty or more years left. Don't laugh; I've done the math, and it's no problem for a raw foodist. At this time in life, I'm able to focus on the satisfaction of living in the moment. I'm also less set in my ways than I was in my early years. I certainly don't consider myself in a category called "the elderly."

If we believe how the media portrays aging, it can sabotage our thinking. We're stereotyped in the media as cranky, feeble, and forgetful. If we watch commercials depicting older people taking prescription drugs to cure just about anything that ails them, we begin to think the drug companies can keep us fit instead of taking our health into our own hands. Commercials tell us we are slower mentally, and if we don't take their drug, we will continue to go downhill. We need to be watchful of the propaganda marketed to seniors.

Our attitude regarding aging is probably one of the most important subjects to address. Mental attitude can make a difference as to whether we *decide* to age well or just accept what we've been told—that our health is failing.

Every person I've met who has a good outlook on aging fares much better than the ones who say, "I'm over the hill," or "I'm at the end of my life," and "Well, this is how it is at my age." We are told only youth is attractive, but I see beautiful people of all ages all over the world. Several months ago I saw a gentleman who is ninety-six jogging on the parkway path at the beach. I met a man who is 110 years young who eats raw food, rubs his body with olive oil, and walks two hours a day, and who said he was thinking about opening a restaurant next year. I saw a woman in her eighties on the parallel bars doing physical maneuvers like she was in her twenties. A man who is 100 recently ran a marathon and finished. A woman whom I recently met at my sister's assisted-living home had the prettiest bright red hair and dressed like a forties movie star. She informed me that she is 100. I told her she was very beautiful, and she said, "Oh, dear, that is just what I needed to hear today." Around the world there are many centenarians and supercentenarians living active lives, chopping wood, making their own meals, and tending their gardens. Although we might be up there in years and might not look as young as we would like to, our faces tell a wonderful story of a life lived: a story of self-esteem, contentment, love, and kindness.

On the opposite side of positive aging are people who see themselves as old. I recently met a woman in her sixties who told me she doesn't really pay attention to how prescription drugs will affect her down the line, as she's already near the end of her life. A few years ago on a trip to France, I met a couple from England who said this would be their last trip out of their own country. I asked why that was, and they answered, "We are sixty, and traveling is just too difficult at our age." I could see they were not in good health.

Surround yourself with the right social circle of friends. When I say "right," here's what I mean: Studies show that habits of others are contagious. If someone drinks, smokes, has a negative attitude, or is morbidly obese, this could influence your actions and attitude. We can choose people to be with who promote a healthier lifestyle and lift our spirits, or we can choose to be around people who have given up on life. A positive, upbeat attitude about our senior years can mean better health and quality of life. With optimism, one can recover quickly from illness or surgery. A pessimistic attitude about our senior years can create a negative outcome in our health.

In senior homes, when residents are told they are frail, they start to become more helpless. I saw this happen to my sister after a fall. The staff at the assisted-living home started taking care of all her needs, pushing her in a wheelchair, bathing and dressing her, and keeping her helpless—mainly so they could charge more for this extra service. As soon as we removed her from this environment to a new senior home, she was up on her own and back to normal. If we don't buy into the negative stereotype about aging, including rocking chairs and sedentary TV watching, we can extend our lives by many good years.

I think we all want to live independently as we age. We don't want to be a burden on family or friends. We would like to live as pain-free as possible and with a sharp mind and sense of humor. Can we trust this to luck? Can we trust this to genes? Can we trust this to our doctors? Taking personal responsibility for our health and well-being is a plan we can trust. With a concentrated effort to eat well, exercise daily, keep our minds active by learning new things, stay positive and joyful about life, love the road map of our face, and be kind and loving, we can extend our lives and enjoy many good medication-free years.

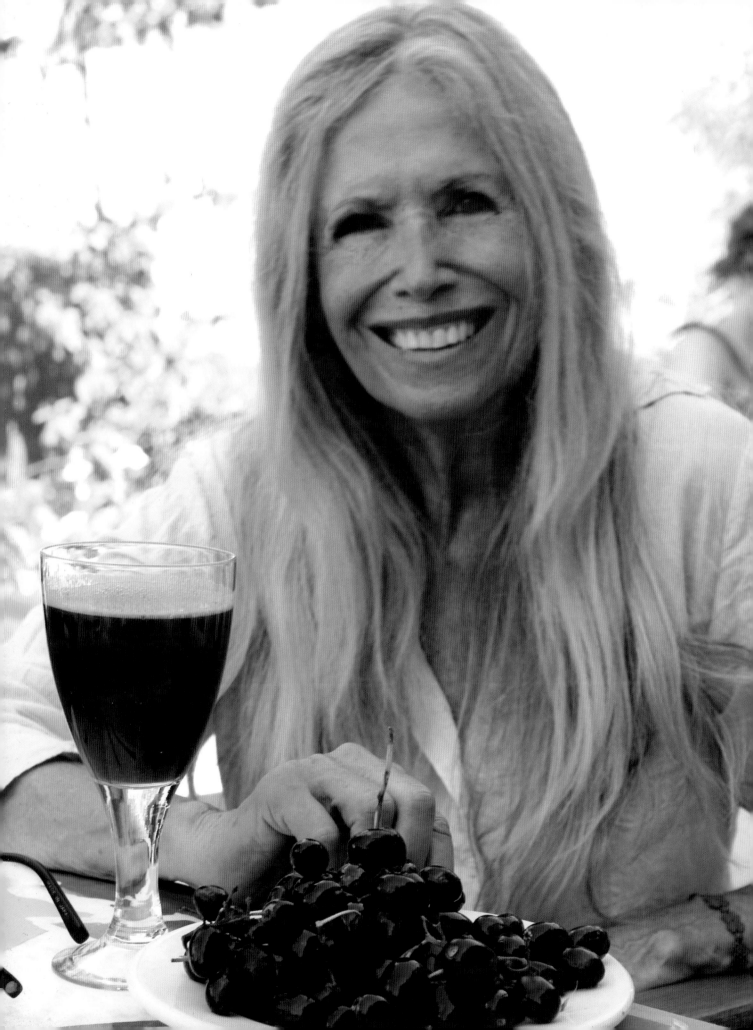

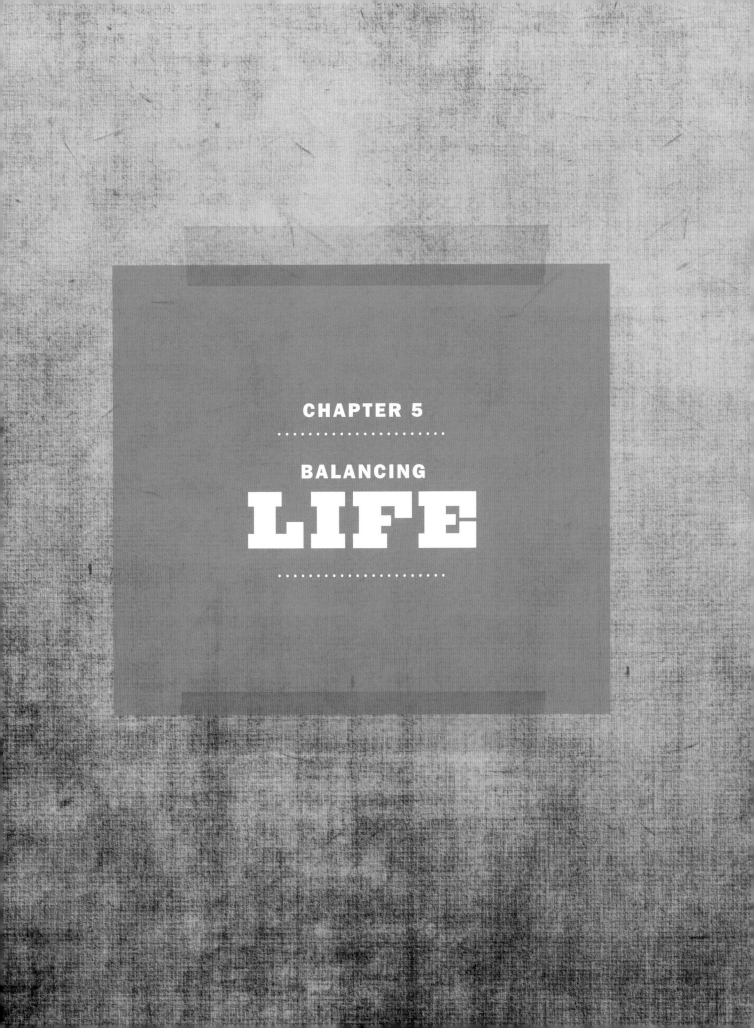

CHAPTER 5

· · · · · · · · · · · · · · · · · · ·

BALANCING
LIFE

· · · · · · · · · · · · · · · · · · ·

so you want to be happy

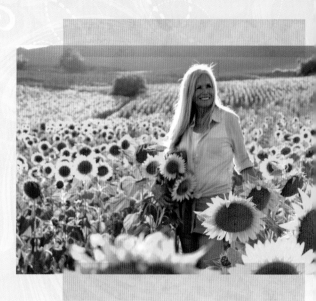

Our mental outlook has much to do with our overall happiness. It's important to maintain balance in our lives. Happiness has little to do with material things but more to do with the quality of our health and relationships.

I recently read that the Himalayan kingdom of Bhutan has introduced a new measurement of national prosperity, focusing on people's well-being rather than economic productivity. They refer to it as "Gross National Happiness" (GNH). They believe the ultimate goal of every human being is happiness, so then it must be the responsibility of the government to create conditions that will enable citizens to pursue this goal.

Success and money may contribute to happiness, but good health, family, friends, love, and laughter have more to do with one's overall happiness. The accumulation of wealth will not lead to happiness. In the big picture, there is an alternative way of living life that is sustainable and meaningful. With each shift we personally make to be more loving and kind, we create happiness for others and ourselves.

Many things contribute to a happier life. Couples can improve their relationships by not getting into arguments and fighting. When both people think they are right, they try to convince the other person why they are right and the other person is wrong. In an argument, we want to be appreciated or acknowledged for what we think is right. We are so set on winning, we become closed to the other person's point of view. There are always two sides to every story. You can both be a little right and a little wrong. In many arguments, one person shuts off and leaves the room, and the issue is never settled. If the argument does continue, it can go on for hours or even days with no end to it. In order for a shift of energy to occur, one person must step outside of his emotions, and drop his ego and urge to defend his own point of view.

Arguing is painful for both parties. The truth is that it's natural to disagree. We will not always see situations the same way others do. There are no two people alike, and no two people can agree on everything all of the time. Sometimes you have to calmly agree to disagree.

If you want a peaceful happy life, you must create it at every turn. Stay healthy, stop defending your point of view, laugh at every opportunity, enjoy each and every moment, stop dwelling on the past or future, be thankful, forgive yourself, forgive others, believe in yourself, be patient, meditate, make someone happy, spend time with children, break a bad habit, smile, spend time in nature, savor time alone, buy yourself or someone else flowers, tell the truth, stay calm, don't be demanding of others or yourself, don't spend all your money, get a good night's sleep, be optimistic, and trust your gut feelings. Remember the days may be long, but the years are short. Be happy; it's contagious!

"A peaceful person attracts peaceful energy."

~ Dr. Wayne Dyer

how's it working for you?

Are you in fantastic physical shape, in a great relationship, successful in business, living in your dream home, and enjoying a second home on some island? Or are you overweight, living at your parents, have a low-paying job and a rundown car, and your mate has just left you for someone else?

What's going on outside us has a lot to do with what's going on inside us. If our lives are not working, then we have to make some changes—mainly changes in the way we think. "If you always do what you've always done, you'll always get what you always got." Some say this quote came from Albert Einstein, but others give credit to Henry Ford or Mark Twain. The origin of the phrase is not as important as the statement itself. If you want to change the results in your life, you must change the way you think. It can be said that life is easier when we are financially secure, our health is good, and our loved ones are at our side—but that doesn't mean we can't still be happy when life hands us some challenges.

Many times we fear and worry about things we think will happen, and in the end they never come to pass. It was all in our mind. Most of us go through difficult issues at one time or another in our lives—financial troubles, trying times, illness, or something that throws us out of balance. However, what determines how we feel about a situation does not necessarily reflect what is happening on the outside but what is happening in our state of mind. For example, one day you might have the best day in the world. You feel great, you exercised, ate well; you laughed and hung out with friends and people you love. You said to yourself, "Life is good." The next day, you wake up and nothing seems to work right. Your self-confidence is low; you pick on yourself about everything—your height, your eye color, your hair, the size of your feet. You look in the mirror and ask, "What am I doing with my life? What's wrong with me?" Why did this change of attitude happen overnight? Did the roof fall in while you were sleeping? Did some gremlin come in and switch bodies with you? How could your life change so drastically overnight? You are the same person you were the day before. You have the same job, the same home, even the same body. You might have eaten poorly the day before or have a chemical imbalance, but your mind is still in control, and it's giving you negative information, just like the day before when it gave you positive information. It's your job to learn how to take the control knob and turn a situation around. If we can see the truth about this overnight switch and realize it is only a moment in time, a moment in the mind, then we can also see all the bright moments even in challenging times. One day of feeling gloomy is natural. Minor ups and downs are part of life, but your mental and spiritual attitude can help you enjoy life even in trying times.

When we look at our lives, there are certain criteria on which we base our happiness: love life, career, financial success, health, social connections, and for some, physical appearance. Are these the things you look to for happiness? Many other people around the world might have a different list of criteria for happiness, such as a roof over their heads, freedom, safety for self and family, food, clean air, education, running water, and electricity.

Everyone's path to happiness is different. It's not that wanting or having good things in life is wrong, but when they are not there, happiness must still go on. All of us, no matter what walk of life we are in, no matter what our situation is, we must take a look at what we can do to find happiness in small places, in everyday occurrences, and around each corner. Small steps can make big changes. Practice happiness; look for good in others and yourself; be grateful for what you have; remember to thank people, especially your friends, loved ones, and people you work with. Say thank you to people who serve you in a restaurant, shop, or market. Everyone can use a smile. Try new things, help a friend, be curious, be kind, get inspired, be inspiring, find your passion, find your purpose, be positive, dream, smile, wake up with a happy thought, create, love, and be loved. Every time you practice something from this list, add something new that will bring pleasure.

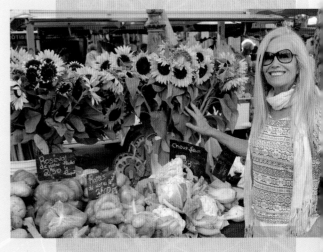

"When you live true to yourself, you inspire others."

~ Mimi Kirk

make your life story interesting

"The principles of true art is not to portray, but to evoke."

~ Jerzy Kosinski

Many years ago, I was strolling in a small town in the South of France with an author friend, Jerzy Kosinski, who wrote, among other works of literature, *The Painted Bird* and *Being There*, which later became a movie. We saw a bride and groom along with their wedding party coming out of a church. It was a beautiful old church, built in the early 1800s, and I felt that we were privy to a very special moment in someone else's life. Jerzy took some photos, and we rushed off to meet several friends for lunch. During the meal in an outdoor café, Jerzy started to tell a story about a woman in a white dress standing in a graveyard with flowers in her hand. He went on with this interesting story, and we were all captivated and spellbound and on the edge of our chairs when I suddenly realized that he was talking about the wedding party we had seen coming out of the church an hour before. I was so amazed that we both saw the exact same occurrence, but Jerzy knew how to pluck out the special and colorful moments and make them mesmerizing. He saw the irony in the fact that the graveyard was positioned next to the path the bride and groom were walking on. He saw the faces of the bride and groom and wedding party and created stories about them. He truly knew how to embellish life and make it interesting. In that very moment, Jerzy taught me to see beyond the obvious and into the essence and spirit of life. We have the choice to make our daily lives interesting or dull. It's all about how we frame each experience. If we see our lives as fascinating adventures, they will be so, and the opposite is also true.

gifts of happiness

In each one of us we hold many gifts. We were born with them, or if you believe in reincarnation, we brought some with us into this lifetime. When things aren't going our way, we forget we have any gifts at all. We lose a loved one or a pet. We lose our job or have a break-up, or we don't quite achieve something we wanted. There are life's ups and downs, and these are the times when it's important look around and remember your special gifts. Gifts can be your own particular talent, or a trait you possess, like being artistic, great with children, a great hostess, a kind person, or anything you particularly like about yourself. Other gifts you can enjoy besides your own when you need a lift can be right in front of you.

1. Take a trip to the beach to watch the tide come in and go out. If you live in the mountains, you can go for a hike in nature. A walk in your local park can be just the ticket. Any time we are in nature, our spirits are lifted. Extend this connected feeling by walking barefoot. It's very grounding.
2. Work in your garden, visit a public garden, or take a walk through a local nursery. Watching vegetables, fruit, and flowers grow can keep us in touch with Mother Nature and all her gifts.
3. Watch a funny movie. Laughter is one of the best medicines. In fact, Norman Cousins, author of *Anatomy of an Illness*, wrote about curing himself from a life-threatening disease by arranging showings of laugh-provoking films and reading humorous books.
4. Taking stock of everyday advantages can also lift your spirits. Having a roof over your head, running water, electricity, and food in your refrigerator are gifts to be grateful for.
5. Run a bath, light a candle, soak in warm bubbly water, and listen to your favorite music.
6. Accepting that all things happen for a reason can help ease almost any issue and is certainly a gift. For example, look at the positive rather then be negative in every situation. There is a reason for everything.

7. Dream. Close your eyes and pretend you are somewhere you love, maybe in another country or relaxing in the sun on your own private island with a good book. Our minds can take us anywhere we want to go. Dreaming and visualizing is healthy.

8. Put down your electronics and catch a sunset. Watching a sunset is one of the best free gifts in life, and it never gets tiresome.

9. Do something you really like but don't usually take the time to do. Get a massage or a facial, go shopping, or sit outside at a café, sip green tea, and people watch.

10. Give something to someone. Giving is a gift.

> "We make a living by what we get. We make a life by what we give."
>
> ~ Winston Churchill

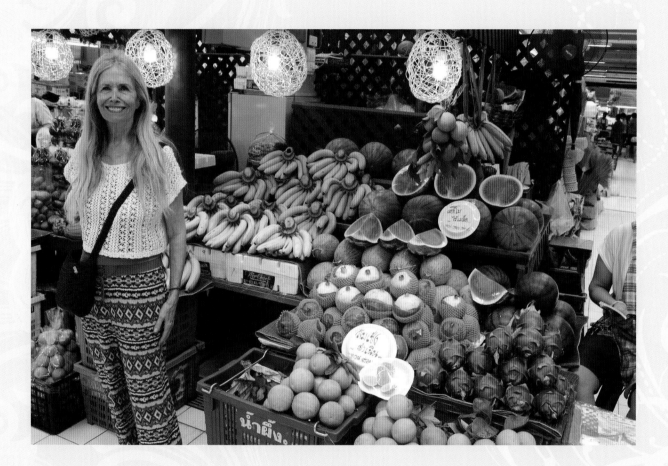

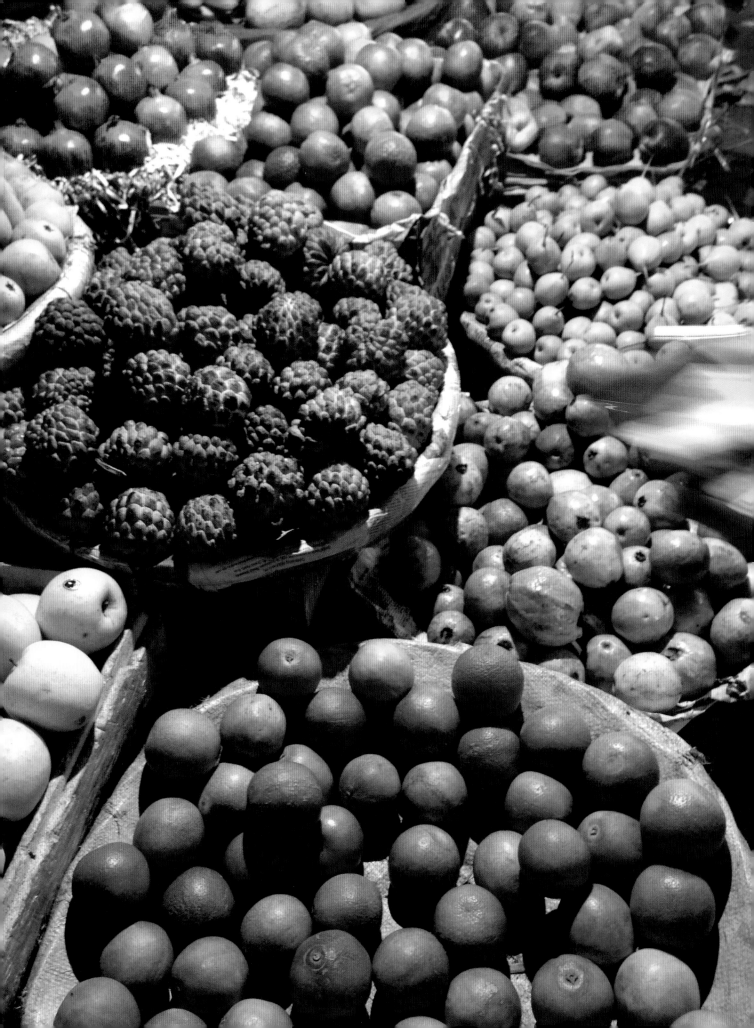

CHAPTER 6

. . . .

RAW FOOD

ESSENTIALS

. . . .

basic ingredients

There are only so many ingredients we can use in preparing raw foods. Some of these you might know. For example, we don't use eggs, which help bind things together, so Irish moss or chia seeds will work just fine. We don't use dairy products, so we make milk and cheese with nuts. All this will become second nature once you start to use new items, and you will enjoy making healthier versions of some of your favorite desserts and cheeses.

When preparing raw foods, there are little twists and turns that differentiate one dish from another. In raw food preparation, many of the same ingredients are used in making breads or desserts, but the tastes are completely different. Some things are savory and others sweet. When first learning how to prepare raw foods, a raw food cookbook is usually necessary, but as soon as you learn the basics, you will create many of your own recipes. Every cook has his or her own taste buds, and I encourage you to use your creativity to make a recipe your own.

When mentioning ingredients in this book, I am referring to organic and raw whenever possible. A couple of ingredients used in raw food preparations are not 100 percent raw. Some people feel fine about using these items, and others decide not to. It's up to you. Nutritional yeast is one of the non-raw items. It gives recipes a cheesy taste, is loaded with vitamin B12, and is healthy. When following a recipe, you can always leave out any ingredients not to your liking.

SWEETENERS

Refined sugar is in almost all processed foods. Refined sugar is known to be responsible for obesity, diabetes, and high blood pressure, to name a few ailments. There are several sweeteners on the market used in raw food preparation, and although some are not consider raw, they are much healthier alternatives. New information continues to be released regarding sweeteners, but in the long run, sugar is sugar and should be used sparingly. I use a variety of sweeteners in my recipes, but I believe each person should decide what is best for his or her own health and taste buds. In most of my recipes I say "sweetener of choice," leaving it up to you to choose from the following:

Lucuma powder is a low glycemic powder, containing antioxidants and carotene. It also contains vitamin B3 and iron. It has a distinctive taste similar to caramel. Lucuma is good to use along with other sweeteners in recipes. It's great in ice cream, smoothies, and desserts.

Maple syrup, although not considered raw, has so many health benefits, it's worth using. It is an excellent source of magnesium and zinc. Maple syrup is good for your heart and immune system. The taste is rich and sweet. I've always been a fan of maple syrup and love the process of tapping a tree, which releases this amazing syrup. It's high on my list of natural wonders. Pure maple syrup is the only way to go. Do not buy maple-flavored syrups. Only pure will contain the benefits.

Blackstrap molasses is made from organic sugar cane. It is not raw, but it's also not stripped of all its nutrients. It supplies calcium, iron, copper, manganese, magnesium, and potassium. Purchase unsulphured molasses, which does not contain processing chemicals.

Coconut nectar has a low glycemic index. It's very thick but not as rich tasting as maple syrup or agave. It is gaining more popularity with many chefs in the raw food world.

Yacon is another of my favorite sweeteners. It is derived from the root of a South American plant. It comes in syrup or powder form. Yacon is a good sugar substitute as it is glucose-free and does not increase blood sugar levels. Yacon tastes a little like caramel.

Raw agave was originally the wonder sweetener in the raw food world, but not anymore. Agave is extracted from the agave cactus plant root, but it is not natural, and recent tests say it's highly refined and contains more fructose than high fructose corn syrup. I admit I still use agave sparingly in some recipes, but I use the clear-color variety whenever possible as claims are made that it is the only true raw agave nectar. Clear agave works well when you are making something for which you do not want to pick up the amber color of other sweeteners. In most of my recipes, I call for "sweetener of choice," but of course I do not mean white sugar or synthetic sweeteners.

Coconut sugar is not considered raw, but many raw food chefs use it because it has a low glycemic index and is unprocessed, unfiltered, unbleached, and contains no preservatives. The texture is granule and very nice to use in some desserts. Sweetening some desserts with this sugar, as with some other sugars I've mentioned, will slightly color the food, as these sugars are brownish.

Stevia is a nonsugar natural herbal sweetener and comes in liquid and powder form. It is used in baking and smoothies. I don't mind this sweetener in some dishes, but in others I detect a slight aftertaste. Powdered stevia is not actually good for vegans, as it contains lactose, a milk product. So if you use this sweetener, be sure to get the liquid form.

Sucanat is derived from sugar cane juice. It's not raw but does not lose its nutrients in manufacturing. Although it is not low in calories like stevia, it contains iron, potassium, calcium, chromium, vitamin A, vitamin B6, and molasses. Sucanat is a better alternative than many other sweeteners.

Xylitol is a natural substance found in fibrous vegetables and fruit as well as corncobs and various woods. It looks like and tastes like sugar but is alkaline-enhancing and has no toxic levels. It's used as a sweetener for diabetics as it metabolizes in the body without using insulin. It's said that xylitol is safe and can help prevent tooth decay; however, keep in mind that it is processed and more than likely made from GMO corn.

Date paste or sugar can be made by blending 1½ cups water and 1 cup dates. Blend until completely smooth. Date paste will last two to four weeks in the refrigerator. If a recipe calls for agave, you will need to double the amount if using date paste. You can make it thin by adding more water, or leave it thick.

Honey is a product that vegans don't use. However, many raw fooders use honey from private sources as opposed to commercial honey. In this way, they feel the bees are not exploited. I've spoken with many conscientious beekeepers who collect their honey in an ethical way. If you purchase honey, a good place to buy is from local farmers markets where you can meet the beekeeper and discuss any concerns. Again, as I mentioned, sweetener is a personal choice. What is right for one person is not right for another.

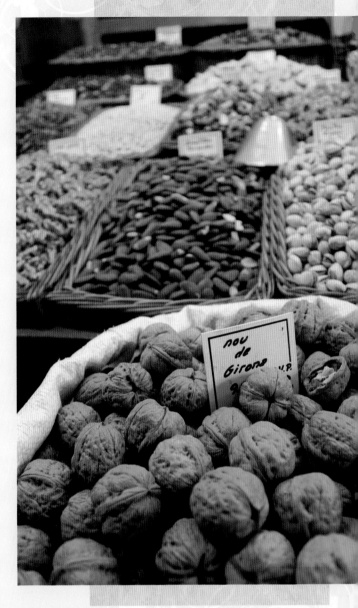

NUTS

Nuts used in raw food preparation are almonds, cashews, hazelnuts, Brazil nuts, pecans, pistachios, pine nuts, and walnuts. You might wonder why most recipes call for soaked nuts. The reason for soaking nuts and seeds is that soaking releases the enzyme toxic inhibitors and increases the vitality contained within the nuts. When nuts are soaked, we can absorb more vital minerals, and they become easier to digest. Flour can be made from nuts and sprouted grains. Processing nuts in a high-powered blender or with a spice or coffee grinder produces fine textured flour. There are several methods to make flour, such as soaking nuts and drying them, or using pulp left over from making nut milks. Nothing can hold back a raw food chef from making delicious desserts and breads.

SEEDS

Flaxseed is rich in omega-3 fatty acids, and high in most of the B vitamins, magnesium, and fiber, just to name a few of the benefits. In raw food preparation, flaxseed is a binder, and when soaked it becomes gelatinous. It is ground or used whole in many recipes and makes great crackers. You can buy flaxseed in dark or light color, depending on what a recipe calls for or your personal preference. To make flax meal, grind seeds in a spice or coffee grinder or high-powered blender. Our bodies absorb flax best in its ground state.

Hemp seeds are from the hemp plant and are full of nutritional value. They contain essential amino acids and fatty acids our bodies need. Like flaxseed, when you purchase hemp seeds, they will have their hulls and shells intact. Like almonds and other nuts, hemp seeds make a great alternative to dairy milk. Along with vitamin E, hemp seeds are full of minerals, proteins, calcium, iron, zinc, and magnesium.

Sunflower and pumpkin seeds are high in iron, protein, calcium, phosphorus, and potassium. Sprinkled on a salad or used to make cheese, they add flavor and crunch to a variety of raw dishes. Ground, they are also good binders.

Chia seeds are commonly used in raw food preparation. Yes, chia seeds, as in Chia Pet. When soaked, chia seeds become gelatinous and are used to help foods bind together. Chia seeds contain many nutrients, such as omega-3, fiber, and protein. Chia seeds make a delicious tapioca-type pudding and can be warmed in almond milk for a delicious breakfast.

FLOURS AND GRAINS

Gluten-free grains can be sprouted for baking and other dishes.

Wild rice sprouting can be done quickly. Place 1 cup rinsed wild rice in a tall mason jar. Fill with filtered water, place the cap on, and give one small turn. Place on the bottom floor of a dehydrator, and dehydrate overnight at 110° F. The rice will be completely sprouted when grains are slightly split and white part is showing. The rice will have swollen, and the jar will be almost full to the top. If by any chance you do not have good sprouting rice, only half of the jar will be full. Try sprouting for a longer time if this occurs. Wild rice is grown in shallow waters in small lakes and slow-flowing streams. Purchase wild-harvested wild rice, not cultivated wild rice. Wild rice is high in protein, amino acids, and dietary fiber. It is low in fat and does not contain gluten. Wild rice is a good source of minerals, B vitamins, thiamin, riboflavin, iron, zinc, magnesium, and manganese. It is a very satisfying component to many raw dishes. Sprouted grains can be used in breads, cookies, crackers, cereal, cakes, and other raw dishes.

Store all types of flour in airtight containers in a refrigerator.

Buckwheat groat flour: Sprout buckwheat in water overnight. Drain and place in a nut filter bag or paint strainer bag. Rinse daily for 4–5 days and let drain. In about 2–3 days you will see a little tail growing. Rinse and spread grains on nonstick dehydrator sheet and dehydrate at 110° F for 6–8 hours or until completely dry. These store well after they are dried and can be used in nut/fruit bars, breads, and other delicious dishes. To make into flour, grind in a spice mill or Vitamix until you have a fine powder. Sift before using. The flour is best stored in a refrigerator or freezer.

Oat groat flour: Rinse oat groats in a strainer, place in a bowl, and cover with water overnight. Place in a nut filter bag, paint strainer bag, or cheesecloth. Rinse 2–3 times a day for 2–3 days. Spread oats on nonstick dehydrator tray and dehydrate at 110° F for 8–10 hours or until completely dry. Grind in a Vitamix or spice grinder. Sift before using. The flour is best stored in a refrigerator or freezer. Enjoy oat groats for breakfast after sprouting; just add almond milk, fruit, and sweetener. On a cold day, you can warm milk and groats in a dehydrator or on the stovetop, being careful not to overheat to keep it raw.

Raw rolled oat flour: 1¼ cup oats will produce 1 cup flour. Soak rolled oats for 4 hours. Spread on a nonstick dehydrator sheet and dehydrate at 110° F for 20 hours or until completely dry. When dry, place in a food processor and grind to a smooth powder. Sift and put any larger pieces left in the sifter in a high-speed blender or spice mill to grind completely. If you use a Vitamix to grind flour, do not put more than 1 cup in at a time or it will not grind properly.

Cashew flour: Cashews are soft and oily. When grinding to flour, place a small amount at a time in a high-speed blender. No soaking and dehydrating is necessary. Do not overprocess because cashews are oily and will turn to butter.

Almond flour is made from the pulp left over from making almond milk. Spread wet pulp on a nonstick dehydrator sheet and dehydrate at 110° F for 24 hours. **Almond meal** is made from almonds soaked overnight then placed on a nonstick dehydrator sheet and dehydrated overnight until completely dry. Grind in a high-speed blender 1 cup at a time, being careful not to overprocess. Sift when ready to use.

Walnut flour is made from soaked and dehydrated walnuts. Soak for 4 hours. Spread on a nonstick dehydrator and dehydrate at 110° F overnight. Grind small amounts at a time in a high-speed blender. Do not overprocess.

SODIUM CONDIMENTS

Salt to taste, as everyone knows his or her own taste buds best.

Himalayan or Celtic sea salt promotes vascular health, unlike typical table salt. We have been told that salt contributes to hypertension, heart problems, and other health issues. However, not all salts are created equal. Table salts are overprocessed sodium chloride and are kiln dried, which removes naturally occurring minerals our bodies need. On the other hand, rock salt and sea salt are sun dried and retain minerals beneficial to our bodies. Use your own discretion when using any salt or salty products.

Tamari is a dark brown, gluten-free liquid made only from soybeans that have undergone a centuries-old method of fermentation.

Miso is a fermented paste made of barley, rice, or soybean. Find unprocessed organic miso in your health food store. Used for centuries in Japanese cooking, it is aged from six months to six years. Miso can be used in any recipe calling for nama shoyu or tamari by just adding water to thin. Miso makes a delicious soup base.

Coconut aminos is a soy-free sauce containing seventeen amino acids. The taste resembles soy sauce, but it is made from raw coconut tree sap and sun-dried sea salt and is naturally aged.

Nama shoyu is a soy sauce produced by fermenting soybeans. It is not for those on a gluten-free diet but is used by many raw food chefs.

Bragg's liquid aminos is a liquid protein made of soybeans and water only. There are no additives, preservatives, chemicals, color agents, or added coloring. It is not fermented or heated and is easily digestible. It contains amino acids in naturally occurring amounts and is gluten-free.

Nori is a toasted seaweed wrapper that is used in Japanese sushi restaurants. Look for raw nori sheets that are not toasted. Nori sheets are a staple in most raw food homes and used for making vegetable wraps. Like all seaweed, they are full of health-giving minerals.

PRODUCTS USED IN RAW FOOD PREPARATION

Cacao butter is used in making desserts. It is a raw product produced without harsh chemicals and has not been refined in any way. It is never heated over 115° F and has antioxidant properties. Raw cacao powder and cacao butter make some of the best chocolate I've ever tasted.

Cacao powder is increasingly being consumed for its health-enhancing properties. It has been used in

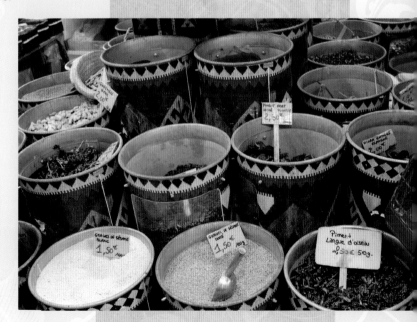

many cultures for thousands of years. Cacao powder is said to enhance physical and mental well-being and contains magnesium, calcium, zinc, iron, copper, potassium, and antioxidants. If you love chocolate, this is the guilt-free kind to use.

Cacao nibs are partially ground cacao beans. They are crunchy and have an intense flavor. Cacao nibs can be used to sprinkle on ice cream, eaten as a snack, or used in baking. Cacao nibs are full of antioxidants and trace minerals like magnesium and iron. In the raw world, many consider cacao nibs a superfood. Since they come directly from the cacao bean, they are partially fermented and low-temperature processed to take out some of the bitterness while keeping in all the nutrients.

Cacao paste is cold-milled whole cacao beans. It can be used just as you would baker's chocolate. Add sweetener and some cacao butter, and make delicious chocolates, dipping sauces, warm chocolate drinks, smoothies, and much more. Cacao paste makes chocolate-making easier. When melted together with cacao butter and warmed in a dehydrator, it naturally tempers chocolate. Tempered chocolate does not have to be refrigerated. Cacao is full of antioxidants, trace minerals, manganese, zinc, copper, iron, chromium, magnesium, and omega-6 fatty acids, which all play an important role in heart health.

Coconut oil is expeller-pressed from the dried flesh of the coconut palm. Free of solvents in the manufacturing process, coconut oil is used in preparing many raw dishes and in smoothies, and is especially tasty in desserts. You can also use coconut oil on your face and body as a moisturizer and in your hair for conditioning. For best quality, purchase the organic, cold-pressed virgin variety.

Sun-dried tomatoes are fresh tomatoes that have been dried to preserve nutrients and vitamins. Because all the sugars get locked in during drying, tomato pieces have a rich-tasting, intense flavor. Dry your own tomatoes when they are in season, or find them already dried on the shelves at your health food store. Some are cut in half and dried and others are in thin strips. Sun-dried tomatoes need to be rehydrated in water before use. I'm not referring to the sun-dried tomatoes packaged in oil, only the dry ones.

Irish moss is a seaweed that grows abundantly along the rocky parts of the Atlantic coast of Europe and North America. It is most commonly purchased dehydrated and is usually light beige in color. It forms a mucilaginous body when soaked in water and is used as a thickening agent for puddings, jams, ice creams, desserts, nut cheeses, and soups. To prepare dried Irish moss, cover ½ cup to 1 cup Irish moss with filtered water. Moss will double to triple in size when soaked. Soak what you think you will need for a two- to three-week period. Soak at least 4–5 hours in filtered water to soften. When the moss turns off-white in color and becomes swollen to double its size, it is ready. Drain, rinse, and pick out any dirt or sand, rinsing well. Cut the moss into small pieces and place them in a blender. The ratio is about 1 cup swollen soaked moss to 1½ cups water. Add water and turn speed to low to start as moss jumps up in your blender. You can turn the speed up as soon as the contents are incorporated and stop jumping. Stop and scrape down the sides periodically, including any pieces that jumped into the lid. Make sure all pieces are well blended and very smooth. Add water as needed, but the mixture should be thick without any lumps or pieces when rubbed between your thumb and forefinger. Paste will last refrigerated for two to three weeks. Irish moss is also known for its healthy content, including calcium, iodine, potassium, and vitamins A, D, E, F, and K. It's a good cure for intestinal disorders, bronchitis, lung problems, and thyroid disorders, to name a few things. Learning how to use Irish moss is a great tool in raw food preparation.

SPROUTING

This is a good source of protein and an excellent way to get nutrients year-round in your own kitchen. The germination process is simple. All you need is a nut filter bag or paint strainer bag or a jar and a piece of cheesecloth. Add good sprouting seeds, including mung, lentil, pea, alfalfa, and radish, to name just a few, and some filtered water, and in a few days you will have sprouts. Soak the seeds overnight, thoroughly rinse a couple of times, and let the water drain out. Rinse three to four times during the day or evening and keep in a dark place in your kitchen. In a couple of days, you will see little "tails" growing from the seeds. In a day or two they will be ready to eat.

Refrigerate in a glass container with paper towel at the bottom. Tails keep growing while refrigerated. Use sprouts on salads or in chili, soups, and smoothies. Sprouts are loaded with vitamins, and the live enzymes are important to your health.

Nutritional yeast is not a raw ingredient but is used in many vegan dishes to obtain a cheesy flavor. It is a reliable food source for vitamin B12 and protein. Nutritional yeast is deactivated yeast and is produced by culturing, harvesting, washing, and drying the yeast. It comes in flake form, is similar in texture to cornmeal, and works well in sauces or soups, on raw pizzas or breads, and in making nut cheese. Nutritional yeast is yellow in color and can be found in a container or the bulk bins at your health food store. Do not confuse it with brewer's yeast.

Lecithin is used as an emulsifying agent in many foods, including breads, crackers, and desserts. With the recent introduction of sunflower lecithin, those avoiding soy products because of allergies or soy's phytoestrogen characteristics can now use an emulsifier that is made using a cold-press system that is raw and chemical-free. You will find the use of lecithin in some breads, pizzas, and dessert recipes. Read labels to be sure you do not buy products with lecithin unless their labels say non-soy and non-GMO. I use Love Raw Foods sunflower lecithin, which can be purchased online or at your health food store.

KITCHEN TOOLS AND EQUIPMENT

When adapting to a raw food lifestyle, you might not have all the equipment mentioned in preparation. Don't let this stop you. In many cases you can substitute. If a recipe calls for dehydration, it may be possible to use an oven. Set to lowest temperature, and leave the door slightly open. As long as you keep a close watch and are careful not to "cook" the food, you can still enjoy a raw meal. You can chop by hand if you don't own a food processor or mandolin slicer. If you don't own a high-powered blender, use the blender you have and strain your drink through cheesecloth if necessary. Having the right tools and equipment makes preparing raw food easier, and when possible, I would recommend investing in good-quality equipment that will last for many years.

High-powered blenders work best. Normal blenders seem to break down and overheat with frequent use. Making smoothies and sauces silky smooth is best done in a high-powered blender. A good blender is more costly than regular blenders, but in the long run, it will outlast five inexpensive ones. I've had my Vitamix for years.

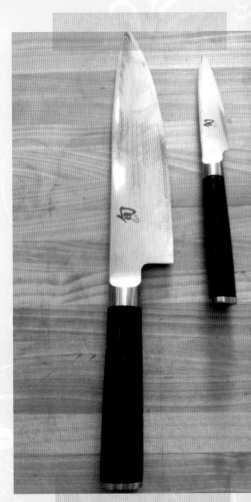

A dehydrator is a staple in a raw food kitchen. You won't need your microwave or oven once you start making raw food, but you will want to own a dehydrator. A stovetop is still used to warm some drinks, warm water for tea, and melt coconut oil or butter. A dehydrator should be on your purchase list if you plan to consume raw foods. You can purchase an inexpensive one, but like many appliances, you will save money in the long run by buying the best equipment.

A citrus juicer is a great kitchen tool to speed up juicing citrus. Lemons, oranges, and grapefruits provide important vitamins. I have lemon and orange trees, so my juicer is an important part of my kitchen. During fruiting season, we juice and freeze lemons so we can have juice all year round.

Food processor: Most kitchens today have a food processor. When you start making raw food dishes, a food processor will become an important tool. It's a great time saver and gives a special texture to many ingredients. Nut butters are delicious when made in a food processor.

A spiral slicer is a kitchen tool that creates spaghetti noodles and other fancy shapes from vegetables. The spiral slicer just so happens to be one of my very favorite kitchen tools. A spiral slicer will turn an ordinary dish into a stunning presentation. I carry a small hand model with me when traveling. Nothing beats zucchini pasta for a quick and delicious meal.

Julienne peeler: Ever wonder how chefs make those perfectly even slices and strips? A Julienne peeler is a handheld kitchen tool that cuts vegetables into thin, even strips. Easy to use, all you do is drag the peeler across vegetables, and you will have sheets of even, small strips. Julienne peelers are fast and relatively safe. Good for fettuccini noodles.

A mandolin slicer is both a professional and a home cook's kitchen tool. Razor-sharp blades make precise uniform slices, which makes food appealing and easy to prepare. There are several different styles of mandolin slicers on the market. I prefer the adjustable platform-type slicer, as I feel I have more control in cutting. Slicing becomes quick, and you will soon want to use it often for professional-looking, even-cut vegetables.

A wire whisk is a stainless-steel tool with a handle and a balloon-type open wire top. It is used for whipping and incorporating air into a mixture, making the texture lighter. It makes blending dressings and sauces a snap. I love having all sizes for different jobs, and I've always loved the way they look.

Ice cream makers are a nice addition to a raw food kitchen. You can whip up a batch of homemade ice cream in no time. Making raw ice cream is a treat, and almost everyone loves ice cream. The best part is you can make dairy-free ice cream without harmful chemicals or fillers.

EQUIPMENT I PERSONALLY USE

Dehydrator: 9-tray Excalibur and 10-tray commercial Weston

Blender: Vitamix, models 5200 and 750 (I'm told Blendtec is also good.)

Vegetable juicer: Omega, model 8006 or VRT330 (I'm told Breville is also good.)

For my last birthday, my boyfriend bought me a Norwalk juicer. It is the only juicer that will keep juice fresh with all its nutrients for 72 hours. The juice is pure and silky thin and tastes better than any juice I've tasted. The Norwalk is very expensive, but it will be the only juicer you will ever have to buy. It's not for everyone, but personally being able to juice enough for a few days is worth the hour I spend juicing. I believe this juicer pays for itself as the Norwalk extracts up to twice the amount of other juicers with the same amount of produce, saving money in the long run. This juicer is highly recommended by the Gerson Institute for people overcoming cancer and other life-threatening diseases.

Spiral slicer: World Cuisine Tri-Blade

Food processor: Cuisinart 14-cup, model DFP-14CHN

Ice cream maker: Cuisinart, model ICE-21

Citrus juicer: Breville, model 800CPXL

Cuisipro Donvier Electronic Yogurt Maker with 8 containers

To make items easy to find, I have put up a page of products I use on my website, www.youngonrawfood.com. Go to "shop" at the top of the menu bar.

herbs, spices, and condiments

While the mainstream medical community only recently recognized spices and herbs as healing sources, spices and herbs have been healing for centuries and are recognized as important treatments in countries around the world. Christopher Columbus and Marco Polo left on journeys to bring these precious spices back home as they were considered as important as gold and jewels. Because of this new passion for flavors from faraway lands, many spice traders built great wealth.

Many of the herbs and spices that give us good flavors are in reality good for us and are medicinal staples for many cultures throughout the world. For example, oregano is loaded with antioxidants, and cinnamon can help balance our blood sugar levels. Herbs and spices are at the very heart of good-tasting food, and a plain dish can be turned into something quite exciting and robust with flavorful herbs and spices. Herbs can cleanse your body of toxins and bring harmony to your spirit. Herbs are used for medicinal, aromatic, and cosmetic purposes. Herbs are made into rejuvenating herbal teas as well as used in aromatherapy. I prefer fresh herbs whenever possible and grow several different varieties in my garden. When fresh is not available, use dried and organic when possible. Dry herbs at the end of the growing season, so you will always have some on hand to spice things up. Organic dried herbs can be purchased at farmers markets, health food stores, or online. You can easily grow your own in pots on a balcony or front porch. The cost of drying or freezing your own fresh herbs is the least expensive and most satisfying way to enjoy them. For freezing, place chopped herbs in olive oil or water and freeze in ice cube trays. They will be ready to use in many dishes, including salads, soups, pastas, and pizzas.

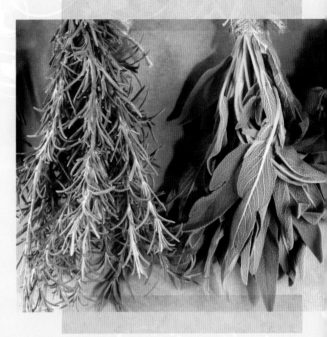

Making your own herbs mixture from fresh herbs is easily done. Fresh herbs can be dried to preserve their quality and flavor. If they are moisture dense, for example, basil, mint, chives, or tarragon, bunch them together at the stem end with a kitchen string or a twist tie. Place the herb bundle in a brown paper bag with the stem end up. Tie the top of the bag and herb bundle close. Poke holes in the bag with a scissor or knife for ventilation. Tie the bag on a hanger and hang in a warm room with air circulation. Wait about two weeks before checking for dryness. When dry, keep a portion of the herbs separate and mix another portion together for use with specific dishes you prepare frequently. Store herbs in glass jars. Do not store near light or above a warm oven or dehydrator. Dried herbs are good for one year. Low-moisture herbs, include oregano, rosemary, thyme, marjoram, and dill, can be easily air dried. Harvest herbs in late summer before it gets cold. Pick in the early morning before they are wilted from the sun. If you are air-drying, tie bunches together at their stem end with a kitchen string or a twist tie and prepare as described with dense herbs above.

The following is a partial list of herbs and spices from around the world. This list will familiarize you with some of the health benefits of these spices and herbs. By and large, herbs are gathered from the leaves of herbaceous (nonwoody) plants, and spices are gathered from fruits, seed, roots, flowers, or bark. For example, cinnamon comes from the dried inner bark of the plant; ginger is a root and comes from under the ground; cayenne pepper comes from seedpods.

Basil provides protection on a cellular level from radiation. It is good for indigestion and bacterial growth. Basil has an anti-inflammatory effect. Basil has a concentration of beta-carotene and helps prevent free radicals from oxidizing cholesterol in the bloodstream. The smell of fresh basil always perks me up and reminds me of Italy. Basil is one of my favorite herbs.

Black pepper is known to have exceptional antioxidant properties that protect us against free radical damage. It inhibits bacterial growth in the intestinal tract and releases digestive enzymes, which help diminish gas. Black pepper also aids in digestion, supports a healthy immune system, and contains a high amount of manganese, vitamin K, and fiber. Black pepper can be used in almost any dish but reduces its wonderful flavor when used in cooked food. Use a pepper mill for freshly ground pepper. It is great in salad dressings and on salads and delicious in nut cheeses.

Chilies are magic, but not everyone likes spicy foods. Not all chilies, however, are hot; some are mild and sweet. They are worth eating for their taste and their health benefits. Chilies can clear your nasal passages. Chilies can increase your metabolism and help burn calories faster, which helps control weight gain. Research claims they have been known to help people with diabetes by helping to control insulin levels after eating. Eating a little chili daily can boost circulation and thins blood, which helps protect against strokes. Chilies are a delicious addition to many international dishes.

Chives are of the onion and garlic family and contain vitamin C, calcium, iron, and potassium. Because of its mild stimulating effect, it improves poor circulation. I like chives in my salads, cheeses, and soups.

Cilantro is an energizing herb that can boost your immune system. It is good for digestion and makes a nice addition to salads and smoothies.

Cinnamon—this bark has bite! Cinnamon has been revered for improved energy and circulation, and for treating colds, coughs, nausea, indigestion, and cramps. Cinnamon is used for headaches and to stabilize blood sugar. It has antifungal properties and has been found to relieve arthritis pain. Cinnamon is delicious in both savory and sweet dishes, and in teas and smoothies.

Coriander is the dry fruit made from cilantro seeds. It has so many benefits. Coriander is known to strengthen the digestive system. It relieves gas and helps release mucus and phlegm in the nose, throat, and bronchial tubes. Coriander can reduce fevers and cool the body. It contains antirheumatic and antiarthritic properties, as it helps excrete extra water from the body. Coriander is used in many European and Asian dishes and is a spice in garam masala and Indian curries.

Cumin dates back to 2000 BC when ancient Greeks and Romans used cumin for medicinal purposes. It is just one of the spices that have been used for thousands of years for its curative and flavor-enhancing qualities. Cumin has been shown to inhibit growth in cancer cells. Cumin calms digestion, reduces cholesterol and pancreatic inflammation, and has antioxidant qualities. Cumin is an aromatic spice and is used in Indian, Spanish, and Middle Eastern dishes. It is delicious in hummus, soups, sauces, and salad dressings.

Curry leaves: Curry is made up of several different spices. Curry leaves or powder have many medicinal properties, including strengthening of the stomach and controlling diarrhea and upset stomach problems. Curry leaves are loaded with antioxidants and are said to promote healthy hair and reduce the graying of hair when eaten or put into oil treatment for scalp and hair. Curry leaves or powder are high in calcium, iron, and phosphorus. They are known to speed up wound recovery and help detoxify the body and are good for eyesight. Curry leaves are dried and ground and used in making curry powders. Curry is used in many Indian and Asian dishes, enhancing their flavor.

Galangal is related to ginger, but its taste is much lighter. Galangal has anti-inflammatory properties that are beneficial in the treatment of arthritis and rheumatoid arthritis. Like ginger, galangal relieves discomfort of nausea and motion sickness. Containing a host of antiaging antioxidants, it can help reduce damage caused by free radicals and other toxins. Galangal improves circulation and contains vitamins A and C. It is a source of iron and sodium and is good for enzyme production. Galangal is used in many Asian foods in the same manner ginger is used.

Garlic cures were once folklore, but now many facts are widely accepted. Many say garlic can lower blood pressure and cholesterol levels. Garlic is high in antioxidants and is antibacterial, helping to kill germs that cause colds and sore throats. I know this from my own experience when my children were young. To avoid giving them antibiotics, I played doctor and made garlic poultices for their chests. I also put the poultices in their socks, something they still talk about today. I gave them garlic tea with honey, and today, their immune systems are strong because they didn't take prescriptions drugs, which doctors eagerly prescribe. Garlic is not actually an herb or spice; it's more in the category of an onion or shallot, so it might be called a vegetable. Garlic is one of my favorite flavorful ingredients to use in food preparation. Whether it's crushed in salad dressing or chopped in vegetables dishes, breads, soups, and sauces . . . however it's used, I absolutely love the taste.

Ginger is great for digestion and upset stomach. It helps with motion and morning sickness. It promotes energy circulation, increased blood flow, and metabolic rate. It is a natural remedy for sore throats, gas pains, and cramps. Popular in Asian and Indian cultures, it is used in many dishes from main courses to desserts. Ginger is a great addition to green smoothie drinks for a little kick.

Lemongrass is shown to have anticancer properties and is also used to treat indigestion. It is being used as an effective insect repellant and fungicide. It is said that drinking 1–4 cups of lemongrass tea a day can relieve bladder disorders, headache, congestion, stomachache, and gas. Lemongrass resembles a hard, dried-looking scallion, but the taste is completely different. It is used in raw Asian soup, Thai noodle sauce, and Thai curries. Working with lemongrass in raw dishes is much different from cooking with it; it takes a little longer for dishes to pick up the flavor. Many times I grind it in the blender with other ingredients for Thai soups and sauces.

Mint: There are many types of mint, and all are good for you. Mint helps digestion—just place a large stem in warm water and let it steep, then sip as a beautiful fresh tea. Mint relaxes the intestines and settles the stomach.

It's good for heartburn and helps support good vision. Mint helps eliminate toxins from the body and helps clean the liver. I use mint in smoothies, deserts, and dressings.

Oregano is good for building immunity and treating bloating and digestion. When used in tea, it has an antiviral decongesting effect. Oregano is one of the most often used herbs in my kitchen.

Paprika is known to boost our metabolism. It contains vitamin C and can aid in blood circulation. As a natural aid to digestion, it promotes the production of saliva by stimulating your salivary glands.

Parsley provides cooling for the liver, clears the eyes, and is a great diuretic. Curly or flat parsley makes one of my favorite simple salads. I always feel energized after eating parsley, and because of its abundance of chlorophyll, it satisfies my craving for greens.

Rosemary: The oils in rosemary help to stimulate brain activity and alertness. This herb is good for your immune system and digestion. I have an abundance of rosemary growing in my garden and cut long stems to keep in a vase on my kitchen windowsill.

Shallots have a host of possibilities for medicinal purposes. Shallots have anti-inflammatory and antiviral benefits and are used as expectorants for relief of colds, bronchitis, and phlegm. They can destroy bacteria in the mouth, relieve headaches, and heal bruises. Shallots are a good detoxifier for the liver and have the ability to thin the blood. Shallots are also used to treat insect bites. Shallots contain calcium, potassium, vitamin C, folic acid, iron, and protein. Shallots are in the onion, garlic, and leek family but are much milder and sweeter. Our bodies digest shallots easier than their counterparts. Use shallots in place of onions. They are mild tasting in salad dressings, sauces, and soups. Slice them thinly on top of a salad or dehydrate slices for a little treat.

Star anise is a beautiful, star-shaped, licorice-tasting spice. Its medicinal properties relieve digestive problems, gas, and nausea. Considered a warming spice, it is known to relieve cold-stagnation in the body. Star anise is also used as a tea for rheumatism. Star anise was used to make Tamiflu, a combatant against the swine flu breakout in 2009, which sent prices around the world soaring. For a hint of sweetness, use star anise in chai, soups, and vegetable dishes.

Tamarind: Like our other spices and herbs, the health properties of tamarind are many. Tamarind helps reduce gas, it's antiviral, and it cures skin infections and rashes. Tamarind helps recovery from colds, colic, diabetes, gallbladder disorder, indigestion, liver problems, nausea, rheumatism, and sore throats, and it is used for dispelling parasites. Tamarind has a lemony, limy, slightly tart taste and is used with sprouted lentils and garbanzo beans. It can be used in chutneys and sauces. Tamarind can be purchased in whole pods, compressed in cellophane bags, or sometimes frozen. To purchase, check out health food stores, Asian, Indian, or Mexican markets, or go online.

Turmeric: The deep golden color alone makes me happy. In many countries, turmeric is an antibacterial agent used as an antiseptic for cuts and bruises. It is also used to cure coughs, colds, and runny noses. Turmeric is recognized as an antioxidant and a liver detoxifier and has shown promise in slowing Alzheimer's. Turmeric is a natural painkiller and may prevent metastases from occurring in certain cancers. It has a mustardy taste, and as a colorant, it gives curries their beautiful yellow/orange blush. Turmeric is the key spice in curries. You will find it in several of my curry dishes.

Sage enhances mental alertness and concentration by increasing oxygen to the brain. Sage contains a great concentration of antioxidants and can be used in a wide variety of dishes. It reminds me of hearty food eaten during fall and winter months. It also makes a soothing tea.

MAKING YOUR OWN HERB AND SPICE MIXTURES

I find it useful to mix some of my herbs together after they are dried to use in frequently made dishes. I also keep some of my dried herbs and spices separate for use with recipes I want to have a more subtle taste and then grind them with a mortar and pestle just before use.

We all have different taste buds. Some like salty or sour, peppery or sweet, savory or bitter. These suggested combinations should be tailored to your particular taste. Use more or less of any herb or spice that suits you. In making any recipe, always adjust herbs and spices to fit your taste buds. Five cloves of garlic may be too much for one person and just right for another. Always go with your instinct.

The following are some of my favorite blends:

Spanish Blend

Spanish herbs pair well with tomato-based sauces, soups, dips, and salsas. For a mixed blend, combine equal amounts of cilantro, cumin, marjoram, oregano, and thyme, a smaller amount of saffron and chili, and an even a smaller amount of bay leaf.

French Blend

A beautiful fragrant French mixture I use quite often is herbes de Provence, which is great in salad dressings, marinades, and soups. For a mixed blend, use a combination consisting of 1 tablespoon each marjoram, tarragon, thyme, chervil, rosemary, and summer savory. Use ½ teaspoon each mint, oregano, and finely chopped bay leaves.

German Blend

German food is rarely spicy. We didn't even find much garlic used in recipes. These common herbs will make a nice mixture for most German dishes. For a mixed blend, use a combination consisting of ½ tablespoon each caraway seed, paprika, chives, dill, marjoram, parsley, thyme, and white pepper. You can also season German food with fresh bay leaves, chives, and borage.

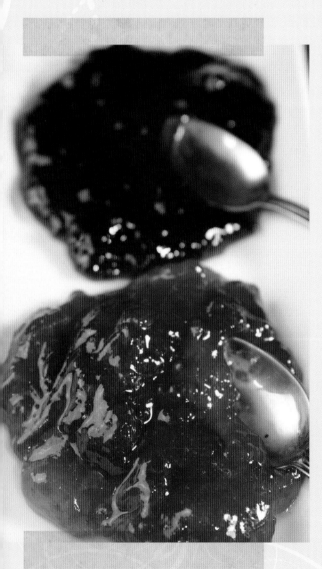

Italian Blend

Italian herbs pair well with tomato-based sauces, breads, soups, salad dressings, stews, and pizzas. For a mixed blend, combine an equal amount of basil, thyme, marjoram, oregano, Italian flat parsley, and a smaller amount of rosemary and sage.

Greek Blend

Greek food is not spicy but very flavorful. Salt is most popular to bring the flavors out of the food, and salt from the sea is of the highest quality. Pepper is on every table to add flavor to the food. No one herb or spice defines Greek food, but the most common ones used include marjoram, sage, thyme, oregano, basil, cloves, rosemary (used sparingly), thyme, mint, fennel, saffron, paprika, allspice, nutmeg, dill, parsley, coriander, bay leaves, parsley, cumin, cinnamon, anise, cardamom, and coriander. You can combine a pinch or so of several herbs to make a blend.

Indian Blend

Specific for Indian cooking would be a garam masala consisting of a mixture of black and white peppercorns, cumin, cloves, cinnamon, cardamom, nutmeg, star anise, coriander seeds, mustard seeds, fennel seeds, ginger, sesame seeds, and turmeric.

Thai Blend

When you mix a small selection of five to seven of the following herbs together, you will achieve a delicious exotic Thai flavor: cilantro, curry leaves, ginger, lemongrass, star anise, Thai basil, fenugreek seeds, cardamom, cloves, cinnamon, coriander, cumin, kaffir lime leaves, turmeric, chilies, peppercorn, mustard seeds, coriander, mint, and tamarind.

Staple Condiments

JAMS

I've been experimenting with jam for some time. Raw crackers or bread with homemade raw almond or pecan butter is delicious, but add a whisper of jam on top and you have a perfect snack or meal. Jams are made with fresh berries, sweetener, and Irish moss or chia seeds used to thicken the mixture. Raw jams taste fresher than conventional jams that are sugar laden and cooked.

STRAWBERRY JAM

2 cups fresh strawberries

3 tablespoons Irish moss or 2 tablespoons chia seeds ground to powder

1–2 tablespoons maple syrup or ½ cup dates, soaked and pitted

1 tablespoon lemon juice

4 tablespoons water

DIRECTIONS

Place dates or sweetener along with water in a high-speed blender and blend to break up dates. Add more water if necessary. Place Irish moss or chia seeds and 1 cup of berries into the blender using low speed, and pulse blend a few times. Add the remaining strawberries, and pulse chop again on low to achieve a slightly chunky texture. Scrape the blender mixture into the bowl, and add lemon juice. Mix with a fork until blended. Taste for sweetness, and adjust if necessary. Refrigerate in an airtight container to firm up for about ½ hour.

RASPBERRY JAM

2 cups fresh raspberries

½ cup Irish moss or 2 tablespoons chia seeds, ground to powder

1–2 tablespoons maple syrup or ½ cup dates, soaked and pitted

1 tablespoon lemon juice

DIRECTIONS

Place dates or sweetener along with water in a high-speed blender and blend to break up dates. Add more water if necessary. Place Irish moss or chia seeds and 1 cup of berries into the blender using low speed, and pulse blend a few times. Add remaining raspberries, and pulse chop again on low to achieve a slightly chunky texture. Scrape the blender mixture into the bowl, and add lemon juice. Mix with a fork until blended. Taste for sweetness, and adjust if necessary. Refrigerate in an airtight container to firm up for about ½ hour.

ORANGE MARMALADE

3 oranges

1–2 tablespoons lemon juice

1 tablespoon lemon zest

1–3 tablespoons maple syrup or sweetener of choice

3 tablespoons Irish moss (see p. 46)

DIRECTIONS

Peel oranges and remove white part. Cut oranges into ⅛-inch slices. Remove seeds after slicing. Stack orange slices cut into quarters. Place the seeded orange slices in a bowl and cover with sweetener. Cut the orange peel into thin small strips. Place in the bowl with orange pieces. Let marinate overnight, stirring occasionally. Place in a glass jar and refrigerate again overnight. Place ⅓ of the orange mixture in a blender along with Irish moss, and quick pulse chop on low 3–4 times, just enough to incorporate. Pour the mixture back into the jar, and add lemon juice. Let the orange mixture sit overnight in a refrigerator to gel before using.

FIG JAM

2 cups fresh figs

3–4 tablespoons Irish moss

1–2 tablespoons maple syrup or sweetener of choice

1 tablespoon lemon juice

1 tablespoon lemon zest

Water as needed

DIRECTIONS

Place moss and figs in blender or food processor, and pulse chop well. Add water if necessary for texture. Add lemon juice and sweetener to taste. Refrigerate to firm up for about ½ hour.

KETCHUP

1 tablespoon cashews, soaked for 2 hours

1 cup sun-dried tomatoes, soaked in water for 30 minutes or until soft

1½ cups tomatoes, seeded and coarsely chopped

1 tablespoon apple cider vinegar

3 tablespoons extra-virgin olive oil

1 clove garlic, chopped

¼ teaspoon Himalayan or Celtic sea salt

2–3 Medjool dates, soaked in water until soft, or sweetener of choice

Water as needed

DIRECTIONS

Place all ingredients except sun-dried tomatoes in a high-powered blender, and blend until smooth. Add the sun-dried tomatoes and water as needed to make a thick, smooth texture. Store in a jar in the refrigerator up to one week.

MUSTARD

¼ cup yellow mustard seeds

¼ cup brown mustard seeds

½ cup apple cider vinegar

1 teaspoons maple syrup, honey, or sweetener of choice

¼ teaspoon turmeric

¼ teaspoon salt

5–6 tablespoons water (as needed)

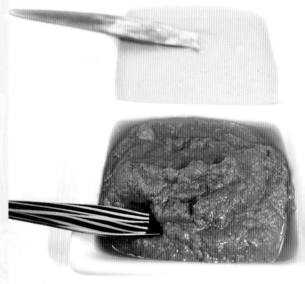

DIRECTIONS

Place mustard seeds in a small bowl. Pour in apple cider vinegar to cover seeds, adding some of the water if necessary. Soak seeds for 24 hours then add all ingredients to a high-speed blender, adding water a little at a time until desired consistency is reached. Taste for sweetness and add more to your liking if necessary. Store in glass jar with lid. Will last 2–3 weeks in refrigerator.

MAYONNAISE

Makes 1 cup

1 cup cashews, soaked for 3–4 hours

2 tablespoons lemon juice

½ tablespoon apple cider

½ tablespoon sweetener of choice

Pinch of salt

¼ teaspoon dry mustard or homemade mustard

½ cup plus 1 tablespoon extra-virgin olive oil

DIRECTIONS

Place all ingredients in a high-powered blender except olive oil. Blend until very smooth. Slowly pour in olive oil while blending until smooth and creamy. Add water if needed. Taste to adjust seasonings. The mixture thickens as it chills in the refrigerator. It will last one week. Mayonnaise can be used as a base for sandwiches, wraps, and dressings.

OLIVE OIL GARLIC BUTTER

Can be spread on raw bread or crackers.

4 tablespoons extra-virgin olive oil

2 pinches Himalayan or Celtic sea salt

1 clove garlic, crushed

DIRECTIONS

Blend all ingredients together and freeze in a small ramekin. Let the mixture sit out just a few moments to make it spreadable, like butter. It can be refrozen.

NUT BUTTERS

Can be made in a food processor or a juicer with a homogenizing blade. In a food processor, use 2 cups nuts and run until nuts are chopped well, about 2 minutes. Turn off the processor for a few minutes to cool down and not overheat. Run again for another 2 minutes, and stop to cool the motor. It will take about 4–5 times until you have nut butter. When the mixture starts to forms a ball, you are almost there. Shut the machine off to cool. This should be your last time as you will see the ball start to break up and dissipate completely, spreading around the bottom of the processor. Now it is finished, and the natural oils have been released. Remove to a bowl, add a little olive or coconut oil and a pinch or two of salt if you like, and store in a closed container in the refrigerator. Each nut reacts slightly differently as far as time goes. The above recipe is for almonds. Cashews, pecans, and walnuts become nut butter more quickly. If you have a juicer that makes nut butters, follow the manufacturer's instructions.

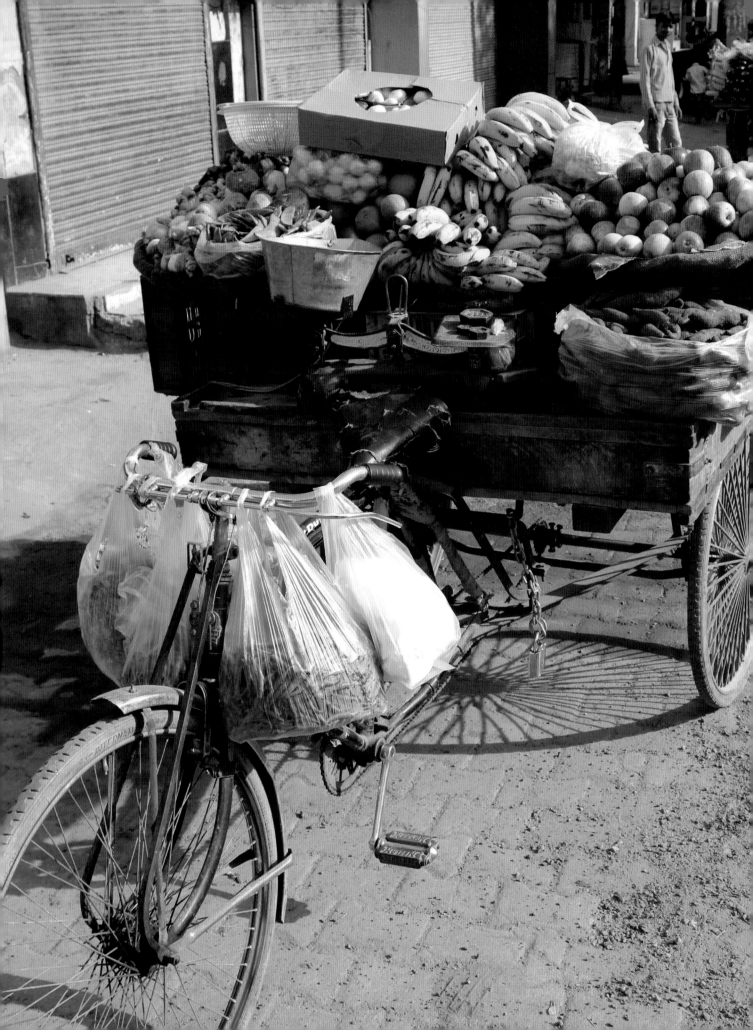

CHAPTER 7

....

SUSTAINABILITY AND SHOPPING

LOCALLY

....

the health of our planet

Travel is beneficial as it expands our awareness of the world around us, but living locally is necessary to support our planet's health. My concern for our environment started in the seventies when I first learned about major environmental issues at the first Earth Day in 1970. Protecting the planet's natural resources was not part of America's agenda at the time, and few of us were aware of industrial pollution with factories spewing pollutants into our air, rivers, and lakes. Gas-guzzling cars were popular and showed signs of status. Reading Rachel Carson's 1962 bestseller, *Silent Spring*, we learned about the dangers of pesticides in our farming, and many of us were just

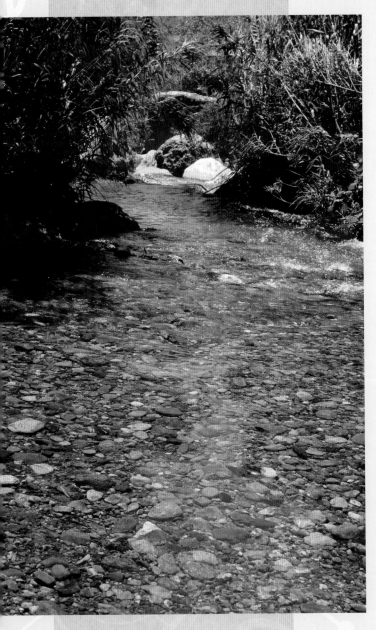

becoming aware of our environmental problems. It was the beginning of eco-activism.

After the first Earth Day in 1970 my children and I started bringing our paper bags back to the market when we shopped to be refilled, or we brought our own box to pack our groceries in. We planted a vegetable garden in our backyard and started composting. As I mentioned in my introduction, I created, edited, and published an environmental newspaper in Los Angeles in 1989 to help educate our community to become more aware of how small daily changes could make a big difference. I would take a bus to work a few days a week even though I had to transfer buses in a not-so-safe neighborhood in the evenings. It just felt like the right thing to do.

Earth Day has now reached global status, and according to Earth Day Network (EDN), a nonprofit organization that coordinates Earth Day activities, there are more than 140 nations now participating. Hundreds of millions of people around the world are now concerned about clean energy. According to EDN, there are more than 5,000 environmental groups today and more than 1 billion people involved in Earth Day worldwide.

What can each of us do to help create a healthier planet and balanced life? One is to decrease our use of petroleum-based products. With more fuel-efficient cars now available and more electric car manufacturers working on bringing us these cars at affordable prices, we now have more choices for the automobile we choose to drive. Public transportation in many countries makes it easy to travel throughout a city. Other ways to make a difference is to purchase organic produce and biodegradable products. You can also lower your carbon footprint and become vegan or go vegetarian once a week. Bring your own shopping bags to the grocery story or farmers market, buy local, stop buying packaged foods, recycle, compost, and purchase recycled paper products and nontoxic plant-based biodegradable cleaning supplies. Buy compact fluorescent light bulbs, wash clothes in warm or cold water, hang your clothes to dry, get a home filtration unit and stop drinking bottled water from all those plastic bottles, turn off lights, adjust your thermostat, and continue to educate yourself on other thing you can do.

Don't waste water. Fresh water is limited. People around the world lack access to clean drinking water, and raw sewage is still in most of the world's water supply. Catch rainwater in a barrel to use on plants, turn the water off while brushing your teeth, take a shorter shower, or don't fill your bathtub up all the way. These are a few ways to bring awareness into your life and help the environment.

organic

While traveling, one becomes more educated and aware of the environmental issues facing our planet. Not everyone is as aware of what is happening to our food. Currently in America and many other countries, we are threatened with genetically modified foods containing GMOs. Not only are manufacturers altering our food, but at the time of this writing, they do not have to identify this on labeling, which leaves us no choice if we want to choose GMO food or not.

Processed foods are in high gear in the United States and growing more rapidly everywhere else in the world. However, many chemicals allowed in foods in America are sill banned in other countries. GMOs were recently approved in Germany for potato crops. They are not intended for human consumption but are developed to produce higher levels of starch for paper manufacturing. The proponents of this claim that using GMO potatoes will save energy, water, and chemicals. Other countries, like Austria and Italy, claim they will outlaw growing GMO potatoes as they feel the latter are a risk to human and animal health as well as the environment.

In the United States, more than 90 percent of soy is now genetically modified. Research claims that our world population will reach 9 billion by 2050, requiring a 70 percent rise in global food production to feed the planet. However, many of us are concerned about destruction to our soil, our health, and our environment by allowing GMOs to enter our food chain. I know I'm certainly concerned and have signed many petitions to stop this from happening.

shopping locally

Shopping at farmers markets is an easy way to make a difference. Depending on where you live in the world, some items must be purchased online, but most of your daily fruits and vegetables can be found locally. Many health food markets carry local produce, and eating what is in season provides us the freshest possible vegetables.

No one is perfect, and not everyone can do everything; just try to do something. We must continue to live our lives and be happy, but we must continue to be aware of the critical environmental issues our planet is facing. We need everyone's help; we need your help. Let's all do something consciously every day to help our environment so we can leave a healthy planet to our children, our children's children, and their children. Remember, small steps generate big results. If you would like some ideas on how you can make a difference, I recommend you check out former President Bill Clinton's website at www.clintonfoundation.org/.

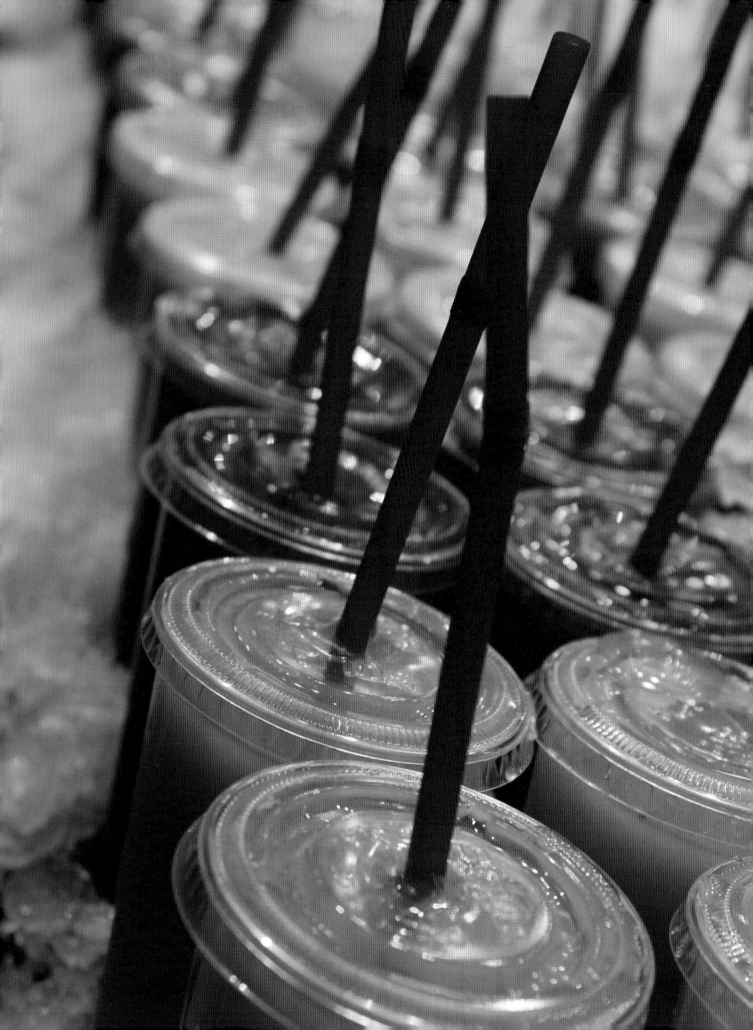

CHAPTER 8

·····················

THE GREEN DRINK

REVOLUTION

·····················

jump-start your morning

Want to improve your health? Have a green drink every day! One green juice or smoothie can have a major impact on your health. One daily green drink may bring you more energy and help lower your weight, blood pressure, and cholesterol. It can help relieve arthritis, poor digestion, and much more. Green drinks may also take years off your physical appearance.

In our fast-paced world, most of us don't take time to consume enough fruit and vegetables daily. Juicing is the best way to get all the nutrients, enzymes, minerals, vitamins, and antioxidants we need. Moreover, juicing releases toxins that get stored in our body from stress and the environment. Toxins can weaken our immune systems and cause diseases. Juicing can rejuvenate our bodies and help heal many diseases. When we eat a fruit or salad, which is so good for us, we do not always absorb all the nutrients because we don't chew our food well enough. When juicing, fiber is broken down so all the nutrients are assimilated and digestible.

Green drinks do not taste yucky as some might think. I promise you they can taste delicious. Once you know the right method and combinations, you will begin to crave juices. With the addition of a little apple or carrot, green drinks taste sweet. If you like a little spice in your drink, a little healthy ginger can do the trick.

There are many delicious combinations, and it's good to consume a variety of greens, vegetables, and fruits, as each contains different nutrients. When you think about it, green drinks must taste good or juice bars would not be popping up in trendsetting cities everywhere around the country, including Los Angeles, New York, Boston, Philadelphia, and Seattle, just to name a few. It just might be the new liquid lunch.

Recently, Starbucks decided to jump on the juice wagon and in March 2012 opened its first Evolution Fresh juice bar chain in Seattle. It also carries vegan and vegetarian food options. By the time you've read this, there will probably be one or two already in your neighborhood. Starbucks is smart to enter the health and wellness industry as it's estimated to be a $5 billion business, and this is only the beginning. The health industry is expected to grow 4 to 8 percent a year. With a thumbs-up from people like Bill Clinton, Gwyneth Paltrow, Jennifer Aniston, and millions of homemakers and business people across the country and around the world, juicing is here to stay.

Fresh vegetable and fruit juices gained popularity many years ago, mainly with vegetarians and vegans drinking them for cleansing and detoxifying, and for a quick healthy meal. In 1990 a smoothie franchise opened. It was originally quite popular but soon received a tainted reputation as its powdered sugary drinks were exposed as less healthful. It still has a going enterprise, but those who are in the know would not drink anything but freshly pressed juiced.

In the early '70s it was difficult to find fresh juices outside the home besides orange and grapefruit. In 1975, David Otto, a friend I've known since I was nineteen, pioneered the first juice store in Los Angeles. He started making vegetable and fruit juices to heal himself and soon wanted to share with others what he learned. His tiny store, Beverly Hills Juice, is located on Beverly Boulevard in West Los Angeles, California, where almost any time of the day you can see a line waiting to get inside to pick up some of his hydraulic-pressed juice or his thick, ice-cold smoothies. In his energetic midseventies, David still goes to local farms and farmers markets to personally choose seasonal organic fruit and vegetables for his store. He's still the hardest working man in the juice business.

Those of us who made our own fresh juice in the early days were dedicated souls, as standard old-model juicers were a chore to clean compared with today's machines, which now have fewer pieces and better extraction.

Since David Otto pioneered his juice bar, there have been hundreds who have followed his lead. For those who don't have time to juice at home or are traveling, the new wave of juice bars offers fresh, hydraulic pressed juices along with some of the convenient grab-and-go prebottled variety. If I purchase a juice, I prefer a small juice bar where an employee presses the juice in front of you or the place has a hydraulic press for bottled juices.

Because the Food and Drug Administration requires pasteurization, all juice found on the shelves of markets and health food stores is processed. Many juice bars offer supplements that can be added to juices for specific needs including, immunity, weight loss, energy, relaxation, minerals, protein, antioxidants, colds, liver cleansing, and longevity. Most offer organic and locally sourced produce. Personally, I think organic is the only way to go.

I love grabbing a juice when I'm out on the road, but making it at home is quite easy, less expensive, and takes only minutes.

I'm happy to see people drinking green juice and take care of their health. I meet men and women around the country who started drinking green drinks after reading *Live Raw*. I get e-mails weekly with success stories and testimonials of weight loss, riddance of disease and medications, and regained health.

Mainstream news and television show are talking about green drinks, raw food, and plant-based diets. They are exposing processed foods. More and more, people are becoming proactive about their health. I believe we are in a Green Drink Revolution. Many men and women who still eat a standard American diet have added a daily green drink to their regimen, and now they are at least getting some necessary nutrients added to their diet.

Years ago, mixing fruit and vegetables in juicing was not accepted. There still is some confusion about combining. If you combine starchy vegetables with fruit, the mixture could cause gas because of fermentation. Dark leafy greens are not starchy vegetables. Greens are in their own category and mix well with anything. In fact, they can help with digestive enzyme secretion. Adding fruit makes a drink sweeter for those starting out and not familiar with green drinks. The idea is to make a drink taste great. Adding fruit is a good way to accomplish that and also to get more nutrients. Berries can punch up a drink and add to your antioxidant intake for the day. Celery is good for helping to maintain normal blood pressure, and cucumbers for hydrating for the skin. Whichever ends up being your favorite, make sure to switch it up for a complete variety of vitamins and minerals.

The following recipes are combinations I've tested. I have my favorites, but I admit my favorite changes every time I come up with a new concoction. I buy what's in season and freeze berries when they are at their peak and best priced. When choosing a recipe, please add any fruits or vegetables you like or subtract any you don't care for. You will soon learn the trick to making a perfect green drink every time.

I covered juicing in *Live Raw*, but I thought I'd repeat portions here to inspire more juicing.

What is the difference between juicing and blending, and which is better? It's all about personal preference. Either one will bring you better health, as juicing and blending are both beneficial. When juicing, you consume a larger amount of condensed vegetables, and when blending fruit and vegetables, water is added to get the blender going to reach the right consistency. Juicing creates a predigested drink, which gives you complete nutrient value without taxing the body. Juicing is recommended when people are healing from illness or disease. Preparing juice can take a little longer than blending, as you might have to cut smaller pieces of fruits and vegetables to fit through a feed tube. Some juicers with larger feed tubes don't require as much cutting.

When you're organized, juicing will only take about fifteen minutes with most juicers. Juice drinks are smoother without any pulp in the drink. Don't be concerned about losing fiber, as the pulp can be used for vegetable patties, crackers, and breads. You will receive as many vitamins as you do with blending.

Blending a drink provides fiber. Blending is a little quicker than juicing, as all fruits and vegetables are placed in the container with less cutting. Liquid is added so the drink will blend together smoothly. I own a Vitamix blender, and I use it more than once a day for soups, sauces, and other dishes. Vitamix might cost more than an average blender, but the motor is strong, and this blender lasts longer than less expensive models. A good blender will make very smooth, enjoyable drink.

Some days I juice, then pour the liquid into my blender and add a frozen banana, mango, or berries to make a thicker and sweeter drink. Alternating juicing and blending is common. Blending also makes it easy to add your favorite superfoods, frozen bananas, and berries.

The following recipes were chosen for taste and compatibility. However, with some recipes I just list ingredients without measurements. This way you can add more of what you like or less of what you don't like. I want you to feel free to use your own judgment, be creative, and don't feel you always have to follow a recipe verbatim.

Learning what works best for you and using your gut instinct is important not only in food preparation but in life as well. Of course, I include plenty of great drink ideas with measurements so you can start experimenting immediately. There will be a green drink listed under Breakfast for each country we visited. If you aren't already drinking your way to health, I am confident you will benefit from this new daily practice.

Drinks will be listed in two categories: juiced and blended. The blended drinks will be broken up into smoothies and shakes. I believe juicing should have at least 60 percent greens and up to 40 percent fruit. Greens are very alkalizing, and those needing to stay away from sugars may increase their percentage of greens.

Sugar-forming fruits can be acidic, so you will want to be sure to add alkaline vegetables and fruits to your drinks. Those with candida, yeast overgrowth, or diabetes should avoid sugars in any form. Severe illnesses should be treated with alkaline diets.

SOME ALKALINE FRUITS

Alfalfa sprouts, artichokes, asparagus, bamboo shoots, beets, broccoli, cabbages, carrots, celery, cauliflower, chard, chicory, corn, cucumber, dill, dulse, eggplant, endive, escarole, garlic, greens, horseradish, Jerusalem artichokes, kale, leeks, lettuce, lima beans, mushrooms, okra, onions, parsley, parsnips, peas, bell peppers, potatoes, pumpkin, radish, romaine lettuce, rutabagas, sauerkraut, spinach, sprouts, squash, string beans, sweet potatoes, turnips, watercress, wax, and yams.

SOME ALKALINE VEGETABLES

Alfalfa sprouts, artichokes, asparagus, bamboo shoots, beets, broccoli, cabbages, carrots, celery, cauliflower, chard, chicory, corn, cucumber, dill, dulse, eggplant, endive, escarole, garlic, greens, horseradish, Jerusalem artichokes, kale, leeks, lettuce, lima beans, mushrooms, okra, onions, parsley, parsnips, peas, bell peppers, potatoes, pumpkin, radish, romaine lettuce, rutabagas, sauerkraut, spinach, sprouts, squash, string beans, sweet potatoes, turnips, watercress, wax, and yams.

JUICE COMBINATIONS

The following drinks are made in a juicer and can also be blended by adding water. Ginger or lemon may be added or subtracted from any drink.

Feel free to add apples or carrots to any of the following combinations to make drinks sweeter and to get added beta-carotene.

1. Spinach, romaine, cucumber, celery, and mint
2. Spinach, green apples, and cucumber
3. Kale, spinach, cilantro, and lemon
4. Dandelion, celery, and cabbage
5. Beet, carrot, apple, and ginger
6. Green apple, spinach, celery, and lime
7. Strawberry, beets, and romaine lettuce
8. Grapefruit, ginger, spinach, and apple
9. Pineapple, orange, carrot, and lime
10. Tomato, carrot, celery, and lime

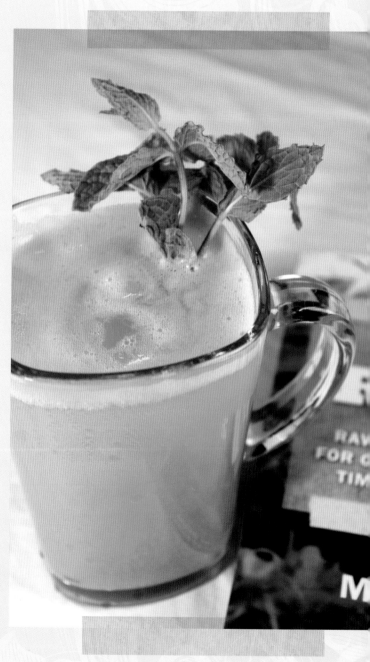

BLENDED COMBINATIONS

Smoothies

Smoothies are blended drinks combining vegetables and fruits and perhaps some superfoods of choice.

1. Mango, banana, spinach, coconut oil, and water
2. Strawberries, banana, pear, young Thai coconut water, and spinach or romaine lettuce
3. Banana, orange juice, mango, and dark leafy greens
4. Blueberries, mango, young Thai coconut water, pumpkin seeds, sunflower seeds, hemp seeds, dark leafy greens, and water as needed
5. Strawberries, dates, cinnamon, spinach, and water
6. Cucumber, kale, parsley, lime, hemp seeds, stevia, mint, water, and small piece of avocado
7. Apple, banana, strawberries, rainbow chard, and water
8. Banana, frozen seedless grapes, apple, celery, dark leafy greens, and water

SHAKE COMBINATIONS

Shakes are thick, creamy drinks made with nut milk or coconut water and fruits. Shakes can also contain greens; a nice handful of greens is always a good thing. Superfoods may be added to shakes.

Using frozen fruits is a good way to add thickness to a drink. Ice may also be added for thickness and so can avocado, which has no taste but is perfect to obtain a creamy thick texture. Avocado supplies good fat and has many health benefits.

NUT MILKS

Almonds, walnuts, pecans, cashews, or Brazil nuts all make delicious nut milks. Hemp seeds also make delicious and nutritious milk. Use milk in smoothies, ice creams, cheeses, gravies, sauces, soups, pudding, and other raw dishes.

Ingredients

1 cup nuts, soaked overnight in water to cover

2 Medjool dates

½ teaspoon vanilla

DIRECTIONS

In the morning, drain, rinse, and place nuts in a high-speed blender. Add 3½ or more cups of pure water to the blender, depending on how thick you want your milk. Add 2 pitted Medjool dates and a dash of vanilla extract or vanilla beans. Blend until smooth. Place a nut bag or paint strainer bag over a bowl and pour the milk into it. Hold the top of the bag with one hand, and with the other squeeze the bottom of the bag until all liquid is strained out. Save almond pulp for cookies and other dishes. Nut pulp may be frozen until ready to use. Refrigerate the milk in an airtight container.

Hemp milk is another good source of protein and makes delicious milk for those who have nut allergies. Follow the directions above.

DELICIOUS SMOOTHIE SUGGESTIONS

1. Almond milk, frozen banana, lucuma, and yacon syrup or coconut nectar
2. Almond milk, frozen banana, dates, maca, and cinnamon

3. Young Thai coconut meat and water, soaking water from goji berries, and pineapple
4. Almond butter, vanilla bean, dates, and water
5. Almond milk, juice carrots, apple, and cinnamon.
6. Pecan milk, young Thai coconut meat and water, cinnamon, sweetener of choice, and water as needed

TASTY ADDITIONS TO SMOOTHIES

Want to make sure your drinks are extra yummy? Need a tasty treat in the afternoon? Time to step it up and add some extra goodness to your smoothie. There are many great organic flavor extracts on the market, including maple, almond, peppermint, vanilla, orange, hazelnut, and coffee. (See p. 209 for organic sources of extracts.) Try adding cacao nib or cacao powder for a powerful lift. Have a go at some spices, for example cinnamon, nutmeg, or cardamom. Nut butters can elevate a drink from good to great. Herbs, including mint, basil, or nettle leaves, will perk up your day, and adding green or ginger tea can give your mouth and body a tingle.

Superfoods

New superfoods seem to pop up weekly. However, all vegetables and fruit can safeguard your body, so why eat superfoods? Superfood is a term many raw foodists use to describe foods that deliver exceptionally high nutrients. One superfood is blueberries, which contain nutrient-rich concentrations of phytochemicals, vitamin C, manganese, and fibers, and are low in calories. Green tea, broccoli, spinach, and tomatoes are considered superfoods. Many believe the new wave of superfoods reach our heart, bones, and muscles faster. Superfoods are grown in pristine soils, on trees, or on bushes, and their intenseness can heal our body quite quickly. The following are some superfoods you might want to experience.

Maca

Maca comes in powdered form and is a highly prized superfood in the Andes. It has great health benefits and helps with hormonal imbalances in both men and women. It can alleviate the discomfort of menstrual cramps, hot flashes, and mood swings. It is rich in fatty acids and sterols, which are known to fight off certain cancers. It's loaded with calcium, potassium, magnesium, and vitamins B1, B2, C, and E. Maca should not be overdone. One should start with a couple of teaspoons and then work up to a tablespoon. Can be used in smoothies, shakes, chocolates, and deserts.

Goji Berries

Because of their rich nutrients, amino acids, beta-carotene, and antioxidants, goji berries are helpful in improving eyesight, strengthening the immune system, preventing aging, and protecting your liver. These little miracle berries also contain minerals and vitamins C, B1, and B2. Claims also say they contain zinc, iron, calcium, selenium, and vitamins E and B6. Goji berries aid in the production of choline, which helps stop free radicals and degeneration of the brain. Choline also protects the arteries and the buildup of plaque. Goji berries can be added to any smoothie or shake. You can soak them in water and use the water in smoothies, or you can eat them like raisins.

Lucuma

Lucuma is a Peruvian fruit. It comes in powdered form and fresh. Lucuma is gluten-free and a source of antioxidants, vitamins, and minerals, and it is a great benefit to the immune system. It has a sweet taste that is similar to caramel. Lucuma is known to provide many trace elements, including sodium, potassium, calcium, phosphorus, and magnesium. Lucuma may repair the skin and have anti-inflammatory and antiaging properties. Use it in smoothies and deserts.

Cacao

Cacao is pure chocolate not laced with sugar. Although cacao has some amazing health benefits and is considered a superfood, it is still a stimulant. Cacao can increase the blood flow to your brain; it is high in antioxidants, which can keep us young, and it contains magnesium, which is good for the heart. Cacao contains iron, zinc, omega-6 fatty acid, vitamin C, and chromium, a trace mineral. Cacao can improve your mood, and it works great to cleanse the digestive system. Cacao is delicious in smoothies, makes the best tasting raw chocolates, and is used in many other desserts.

Probiotics

Probiotics are very important to our health. Probiotics are living beneficial microorganisms that are good for our digestive tract and help keep the bad bacteria away. They produce antibodies, which strengthen our immune system. They build a barrier against infection. Probiotics produce B vitamins and ward off anemia caused by B deficiencies. They can help us maintain healthier skin and nervous systems. Use probiotics in making cheese, and add them to some smoothies or coconut yogurt.

Blue-Green Algae

Blue-green algae can be found in powder, capsules, and pill form. It's a microscopic plant found in lakes. Spirulina falls into the same category as blue-green algae. This amazing green contains vitamins C and E, beta-carotene, minerals, protein, and folate. Mainly, blue-green algae are rich in chlorophyll. Blue-green algae are found to prevent and cure many diseases, such as asthma, allergies, depression, fatigue, digestive issues, heart problems, and attention deficit disorder. They are also used for weight loss and to treat memory loss. Blue-green algae are used in smoothies when detoxifying.

Aloe Vera

Aloe is a decorative succulent plant. It is used as a medicinal herb both externally and internally and is known to have been in existence for more than 4,000 years. In the Middle Ages, the Romans and Greeks used aloe vera to treat wounds and relieve digestive discomforts. It's used for kitchen burns and to strengthen the immune system.

When my children were growing up, I always had a little potted plant of aloe vera just outside the kitchen door. Researchers of aloe make some strong claims for its amazing healing properties. There have been studies indicating aloe has been used to treat type 2 diabetes and inhibit tumor growth, and has a major antihyperglycemic effect. Aloe vera is sold in many forms today, including liquid and capsule. If you can get your hands on a fresh leaf, you can split it open down the center with a sharp knife and scrape the sticky gel-like substance from the center. Handle with care, as the spines down the sides can be a little tricky. A small amount of gel can be used in smoothies. If you overdo it, look forward to a quick trip to the bathroom. I suppose if you are eating raw, you do not have to worry about cooking burns, but it's good to have aloe on hand for any wound.

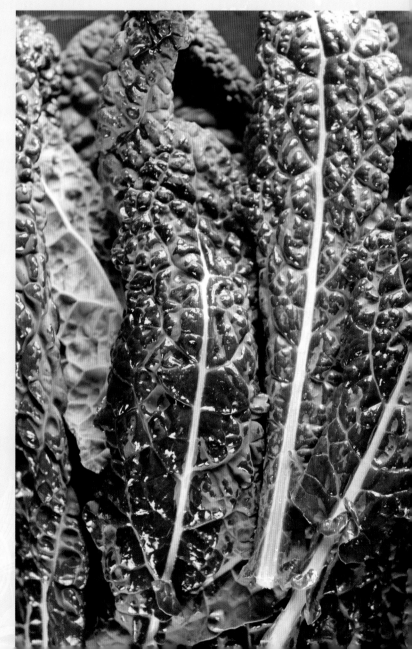

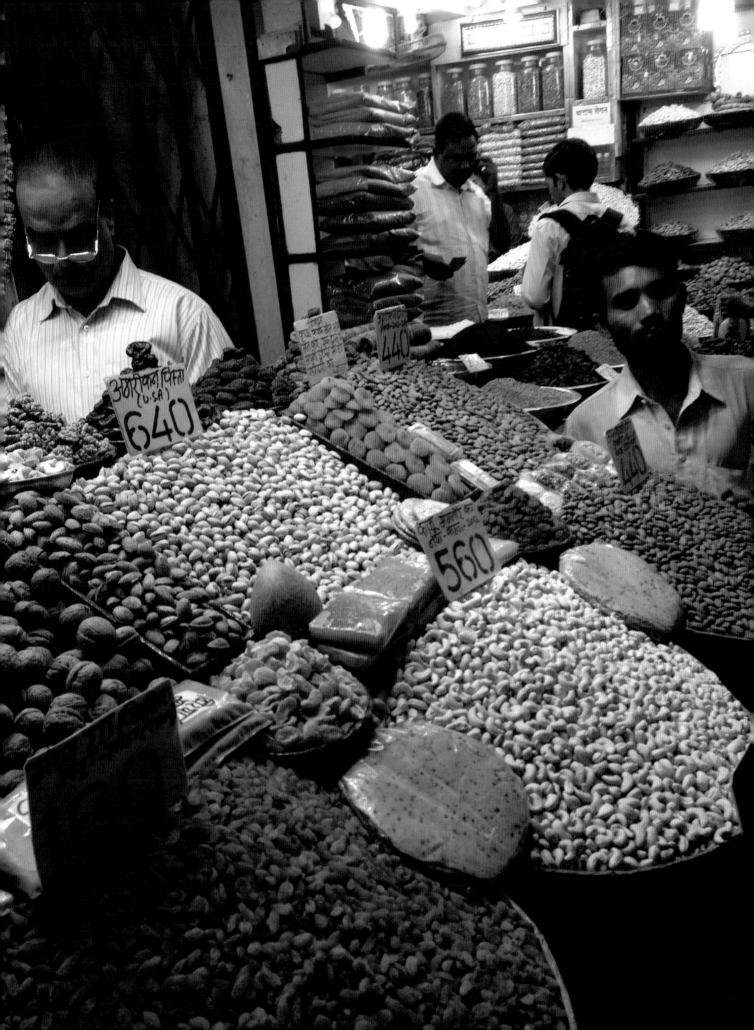

CHAPTER 9

....

RAW FOOD RECIPES FROM AROUND THE

WORLD

....

I hope my neighbors around the world will take kindly to my revising some of their classic dishes into raw ones. It's because I admire and appreciate fine cooking that I have taken the liberty to find ways to still enjoy international food while eating a raw vegan diet. With all due respect, I've expressed my interpretation of some of my favorite dishes from the countries I visited. There were so many great recipes developed in the process, and I really had to pick and choose which ones to include.

The following recipes are in order of the places we traveled. We arrived in Barcelona, Spain, on June 23, 2012, and continued on to France, Germany, Italy, and Greece. We then took a short break home to test recipes and finish up some writing, and a little over a month later we left for India and Bangkok to finalize recipes and photos.

MY RECIPE FOR LIFE

- A ton of love
- A gallon of kindness
- 10 pounds of positivity
- Several cups of generosity
- Sweetness to taste
- Enough confidence to hold it all together

DIRECTIONS

Marinate for ten or more decades, garnish with a smile, and enjoy.

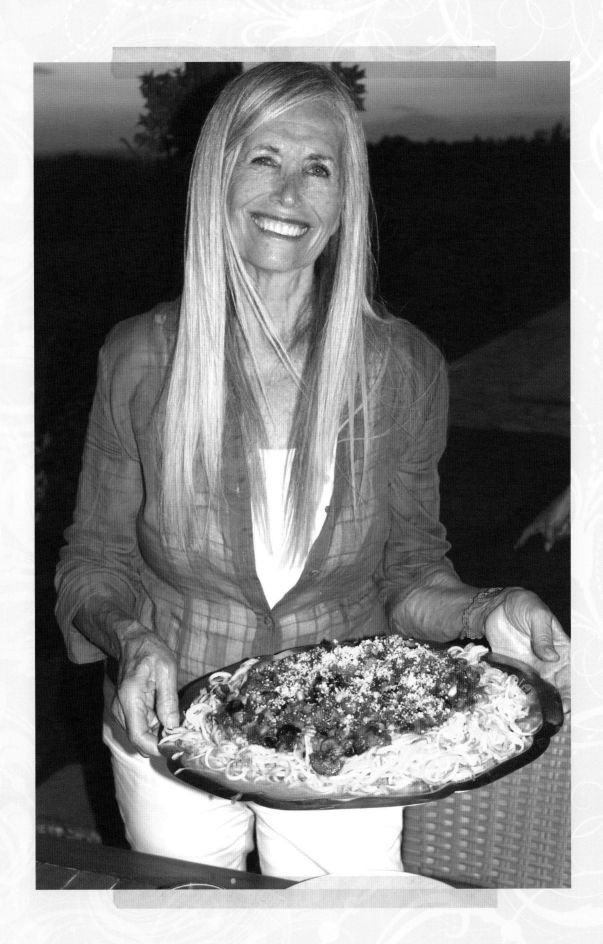

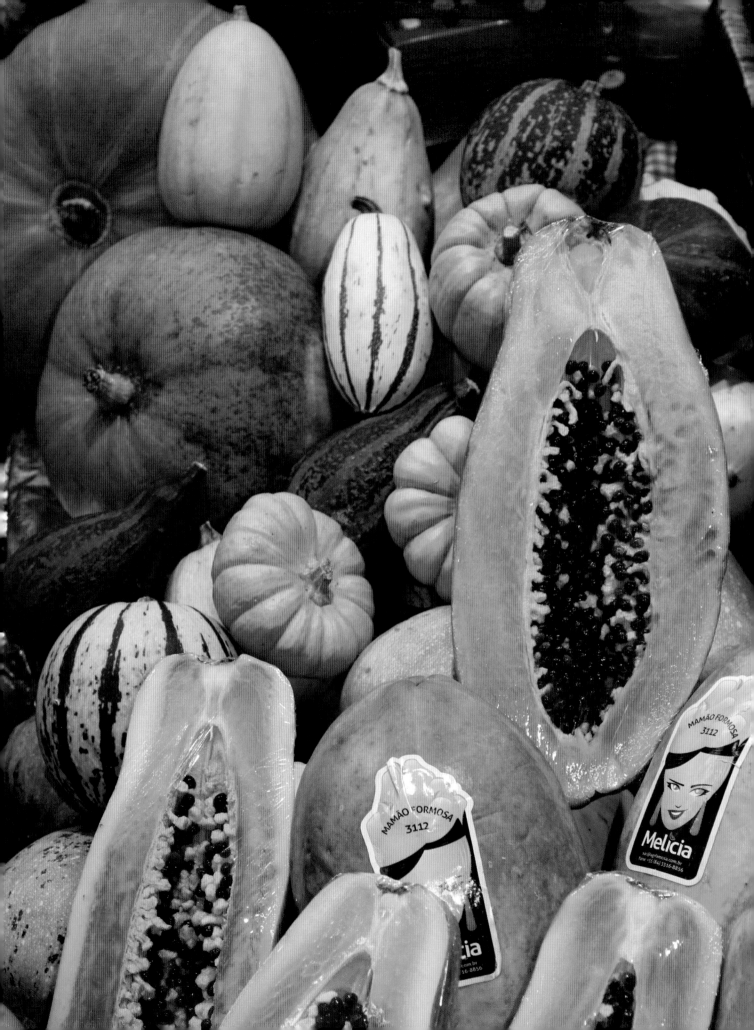

CHAPTER 10

· · · · · · · · · · · · · · · · · · ·

RAW CUISINE—TASTE OF
SPAIN

· · · · · · · · · · · · · · · · · · ·

Ever since I saw the television special called *Spain... On the Road Again*, with Mario Batali and Gwyneth Paltrow, I've wanted to visit this beautiful country. Batali and Paltrow toured Spain to eat, write a cookbook, and produce a television series. Even though I don't eat the array of food they consumed on their trip, I knew I could enjoy all the fresh and succulent fruits and veggies Spain had to offer. The show enticed me with the beauty of the country and friendliness of its people. The architecture alone is enough to draw anyone to Barcelona. Antoni Gaudí's work, including the Sagrada Família church, and Lluís Domènech i Montaner's unique work make Barcelona a rich cultural city and a major tourist destination. People can find almost anything they are looking for in this city; fashion, entertainment, science, sports, and great food all make Barcelona a growing tourist and financial center.

I did a little research to see where we wanted to spend our time while in Barcelona, and we made the rounds, covering many places in a short time. We stayed in the business section at Hotel Diagonal Zero and could not have asked for anything more. Our room was beautifully appointed, comfortable, with amazing views. We had deluxe accommodations with use of spa, pool, and rooftop garden, and a breakfast with enough perfectly ripe fruit to make any raw foodist happy. The location was just a four-minute walk from the metro, which enabled us to get anywhere in the city in just minutes.

I contacted the only raw chef I could find in Barcelona, Chef Christine Mayr of Crua Gourmet Cuisine, who trained at Living Light Institute in Northern California. Chef Christine invited me to present a demonstration of one of my recipes at a raw food class she was giving. The class was in Spanish, so she translated my Caesar salad recipe while I spoke. I was happy to see that my dish was a big hit, as every recipe Christine demonstrated from soup to desert was simply delicious. The class was held in a beautiful art gallery that had a lovely little kitchen. Christine's boyfriend, Frank Capellades, a talented graphic designer and branding expert, was busy in the kitchen plating food, washing veggies, and being her right-hand man for the evening.

Christine and I immediately hit if off as we both share the love of good quality ingredients, deliciously prepared, and the art of plating food to make a beautiful presentation. I now include her in my list of favorite top raw food chefs, and both she and Frank are good friends. Find out more about Christine at wwwcruagourmetcuisine.com.

The following day, Christine picked us up at our hotel for a day of fun, sightseeing, and food talk. I learned from her that raw food has not really taken off yet in Spain. There are plenty of vegetarian and vegan choices, and although one can find raw selections on a menu, they are not intentionally put there for vegetarians or vegans and are mostly salads. Catalonians like to stick to their traditional foods and don't understand raw food preparation just yet. Christine has her work cut out for her. She writes about raw food for a local magazine, caters, works as a private chef for a family, stays busy giving monthly food preparation classes, and lectures any chance she gets. I have no doubt she is changing people's minds about eating raw food everywhere she goes.

Christine introduced me to her friend Mandy Keillor, who owns and operates Pilates Studio Australia. Mandy trains her clients on the original Pilates machine that became famous when it was created for helping dancers many years ago. Mandy's studio is absolutely breathtaking. We took an iron-door

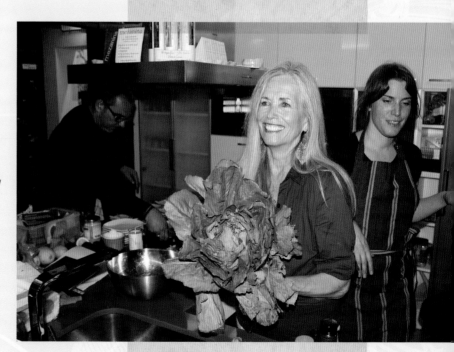

elevator to her studio level and walked into the most serene atmosphere. Mandy is the author of *Detox Guide: A Simple Guide to Purify Your Body at Home in 14 Days* as well as the amazing iPhone app *Face Pilates*. Mandy's line of natural products is one of the very best I've ever tried. If you venture to Barcelona, put a class with her at the top of your to-do list. Pilates can rejuvenate the body at any age. It was very rewarding to be in Barcelona and find people like Christine and Mandy, who are bringing conscious living and health to Spain.

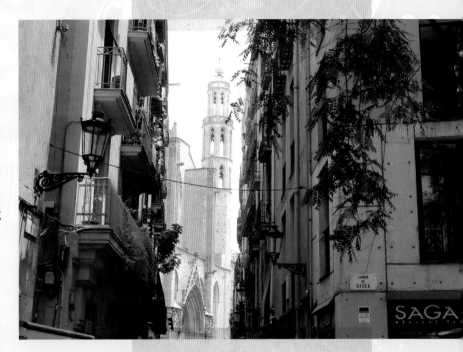

I read about farmers markets in Barcelona and was really looking forward to the famous Mercat de Sant Josep de a Boqueria, simply referred to as La Boqueria, (pronounced la bow-KA-ree-ah), one of the oldest and largest markets in Spain. The first mention of La Boqueria dates back to 1217. La Boqueria is a large permanent indoor market in Catalunya, which connects to La Rambla, a main tourist street in Barcelona Catalonia. At La Boqueria, we found stall after stall of fruits and vegetables, including several organic stands. Fresh juice of every color was sitting in to-go containers in mounds of shaved ice. I later learned that many vendors put sugar in their drinks, so you have to ask if you want to find pure juice. There were piles of freshly cut-up fruit in take-away containers. I could live in Barcelona for this marketplace alone. Beautiful raw nuts and spices more than tempted me, and we bought snacks for the train. It's not that one can find organic everywhere, but after speaking to several farmers, they told me they don't spray their products.

There were a great number of nonvegan foods at the market from which I had to avert my eyes, but there was plenty of produce to enjoy delicious raw meals and stay healthy while in Spain. Any fresh, plant-based food is far better than eating processed foods while traveling. I believe the people of Spain understand the notion of fresh whole foods, and many shop daily to prepare family meals.

We also found a couple of vegetarian/vegan restaurants, which surprised me, as Spain is not what I'd call a vegetarian-conscious country. We ate at Veggie Gardens and at Juicy Jones, both vegan restaurants, and had extremely delicious, satisfying salads with a variety of fresh veggies. Cat Bar is also starting to add more vegan and raw foods.

spanish herbs and spices of spain

America was discovered by accident while Christopher Columbus was sailing in search of jewels and spices. It's no wonder that King Ferdinand and Queen Isabella of Spain funded the sailing ships for this Italian. Spaniards have always loved their spices as much as they do their gold. Spaniards have cultivated herbs and spices for thousands of years, and you will never taste a bland dish in Spain. The wonderful thing about Spanish cooking is the freshly prepared food with subtly flavored spices. An intuitive pinch of this and an artful dash of that is the way food is brought to life—it's not spicy but always flavorful with rich aroma and color.

Paprika gives dishes a beautiful tint and can be found sweet, smoked, or picante. Cayenne is used delicately, and garlic is everywhere, even found hanging in shop doorways.

What would a Spanish dish like paella be without the perfume scent of saffron, with its beautiful orange-red color that diffuses into a golden yellow? Saffron has a complex taste like a bitter honey and a little alfalfa thrown in—used properly, it adds a special, delightful taste to many dishes. Just a pinch goes a long way, which is a good thing since saffron has always been one of the most expensive spices on the market. I have a new understanding about saffron after learning how difficult it is to harvest. One flower produces only three threads. Over 150 flower heads are needed to make one gram of dried saffron threads.

Other popular spices and herbs used in Spanish cooking are vanilla, cinnamon, cloves, and nutmeg. Mint, parsley, rosemary, basil, thyme, oregano, and tarragon are chopped finely and used fresh. Bay leaf, coriander, cardamom, and caraway are also popular for bringing a unique taste to a dish. No Spanish kitchen is without good quality salt and pepper to season most dishes.

The Catalan diet is part of the Mediterranean diet. Although there are three meals a day, I noticed that breakfast was very light, consisting of fruit or fruit juice and coffee and a possibly a small pastry. Lunch was the heaviest meal of the day, and dinner was eaten quite late and accompanied by wine.

Buen Provecho (Enjoy Your Meal)

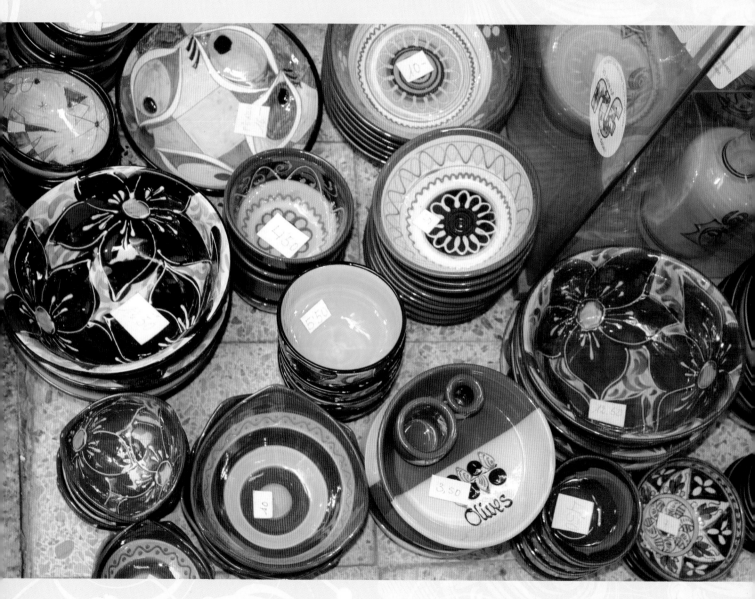

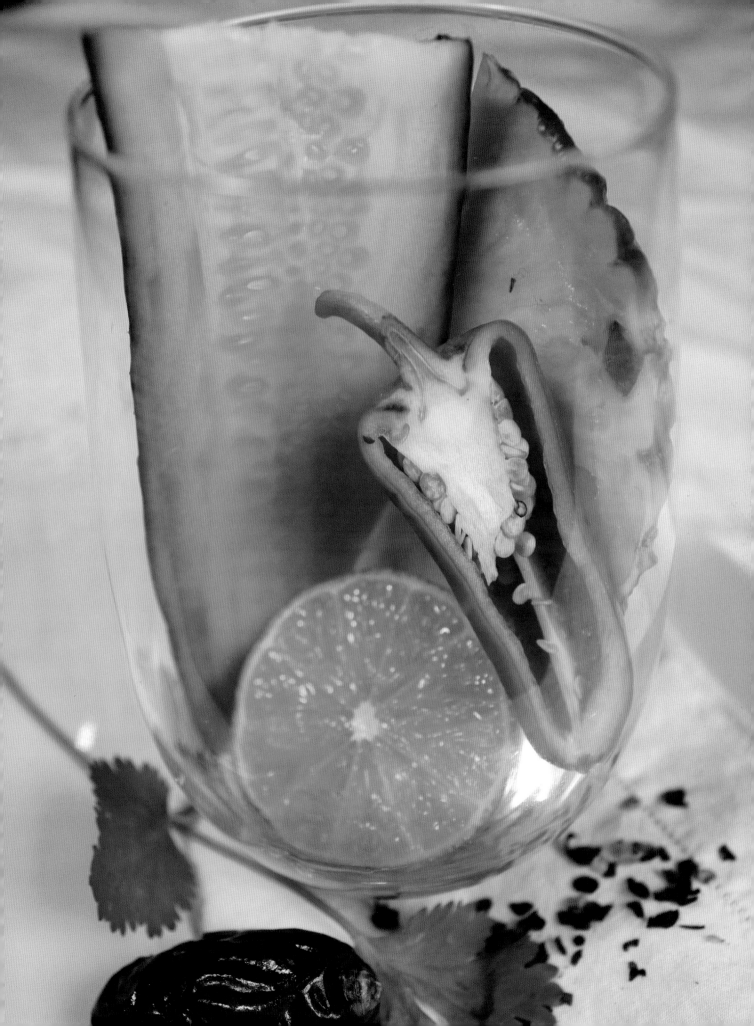

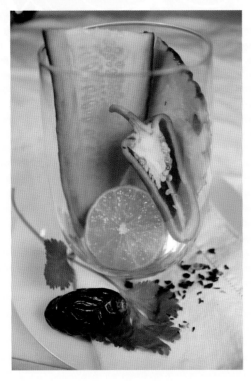

Breakfast (El Desayuno)

SPANISH GREEN DRINK WITH A KICK

A simple drink can be a sufficient breakfast.

1 cup pineapple

1 cucumber

1 lime, juiced

½ lime zest

1 small piece of jalapeño—if you like spice (optional)

1½ cups water

2 teaspoons maple syrup, dates, or sweetener of choice to taste

DIRECTIONS

Blend in a high-speed blender until smooth. Pour over ice, and use zest to garnish top.

Una Mezcla of Berries

Only buy organic berries, as berries hold the greatest amount of pesticides when purchased conventionally.

1 cup mixed berries, strawberries, blackberries, raspberries, and blueberries

¼ cup orange juice

¼ cup lemon juice

DIRECTIONS

Mix juices with a little sweetener of choice and pour over berries. Garnish with chopped mint leaves.

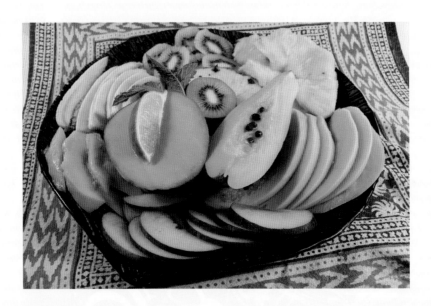

Una Mezcla of Fruits

Una Mezcla of Fresh Market Fruits *(una mezcla = a mixture or assortment) This beautiful and colorful dish is always unique and never the same. What's fresh at the market is what is used for the recipe.*

Mango, thinly sliced	Pineapple, thinly sliced
Papaya, thinly sliced	½ cup orange juice
Banana, thinly sliced	¼ cup lime juice

DIRECTIONS

Arrange alternating fruit in a fan around the plate. Combine a mixture of orange and lime juice, add sweetener of choice, and garnish with chopped mint leaves.

Mini Churros with Cinnamon and Coconut Sugar

Preparation is necessary to sprout the buckwheat, around 2–3 days

1 cup buckwheat, sprouted	4 tablespoons coconut sugar
2 cups cashews, soaked for 4 hours	1 tablespoon cinnamon
½ cup young Thai coconut meat or psyllium	1 teaspoon vanilla powder or extract
1 cup Medjool dates, soaked until soft	½ cup water

DIRECTIONS

Place cashews, buckwheat, coconut meat, and dates in a bowl and combine. Run ingredients through a blank plate of your juicer, or blend in a high-speed blender and add just enough water to make a thick, smooth dough. If using a juicer, run through twice to achieve a smooth batter. It's nice to have a churro maker, and you can purchase one for around $20 if you decide to put this recipe on your list of favorites. In the meantime, use a pastry bag. There is a plastic piece that gets dropped in the pastry bag that the decorating tips fit into, and this is what I used for shaping the churros. The opening on this plastic tip will be the largest one that comes with the set. Fill the piping bag with dough, leaving enough room at the top of the bag to get a good grip to squeeze the dough onto nonstick dehydrator sheets. Make strips about 4–5 inches long. Dehydrate for 3 hours at 110° F, then flip onto mesh screen and dehydrate for another 10 hours or until the texture you desire is reached. Mix cinnamon and coconut sugar or xylitol on a large plate, and combine well. When churros are finished, brush with melted coconut oil and roll in cinnamon/sugar mixture to coat. Serve warm or at room temperature.

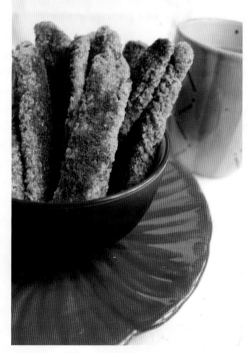

TIP { If you don't have a pastry bag, use a Ziploc bag with an angled cut at the bottom end to squeeze mixture into proper shape.

Lunch (La Comida) (la comida = midday meal)

CEVICHE VEGANO

- 3 medium tomatoes, seeded and diced
- ½ small red onion, finely chopped
- ½ bunch cilantro leaves, chopped
- 1 jalapeño, seeded and diced (or to taste)
- Juice of 2 limes
- 2 green onions, chopped
- ½ English or 2–3 Persian cucumbers, peeled and diced
- ½ green bell pepper, diced
- 1 tablespoon extra-virgin olive oil
- 1 clove garlic, crushed
- Pinch of chili powder
- Himalayan salt to taste
- Freshly milled pepper to taste
- 1 large avocado, cut in long wedges for topping

DIRECTIONS

Mix tomatoes, ½ of the onion, and ½ of the cilantro together in a small bowl. Reserving 1 teaspoon for topping each serving, place remaining tomato mixture in glasses, such as a highball glass. Mix remaining ingredients, except avocado, in a large bowl. Toss gently. Place on top of tomato mixture, and drizzle a little olive oil on top. Finish off with remaining tomato mixture. Place wedge of avocado on top of each glass to finish off the dish, and serve with a small slice of lime on the side. Chill for 1–2 hours before serving.

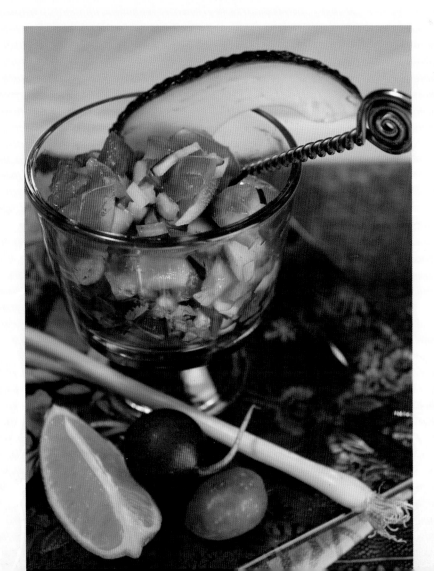

Spanish Gazpacho (chilled tomato soup with assorted vegetables)

This soup will inspire your creativity. Spices are all up to your taste buds. During summer months, I could eat this soup daily; it's simple to make, yet so deliciously satisfying and healthy.

4 large ripe tomatoes, cut in quarters, seeds removed

1 small yellow bell pepper, broken in pieces

1 small sweet red pepper, broken in pieces

1 large English cucumber, cut in chunks

¼ cup shallots, cut in pieces

1 apple, cut into chunks, seeds removed

2 tablespoons good-quality extra-virgin olive oil

1–2 cloves garlic, crushed

1–2 dates

½ bunch mint leaves

Juice from ½ lime

Himalayan salt to taste

Freshly milled pepper to taste

Water as needed to reach desired consistency

Garnish with chopped scallions, thinly sliced radishes, and avocado

DIRECTIONS

Use a blender or food processor and chop all vegetables to desired texture. I like mine just a little chunky but well incorporated. If you prefer a thinner texture, add a little water or blend for a longer time. Mixture is best if chilled before serving. When ready to serve, place in bowls and garnish with scallions and avocado.

TIP { Spice it up with chili flakes or chili oil.

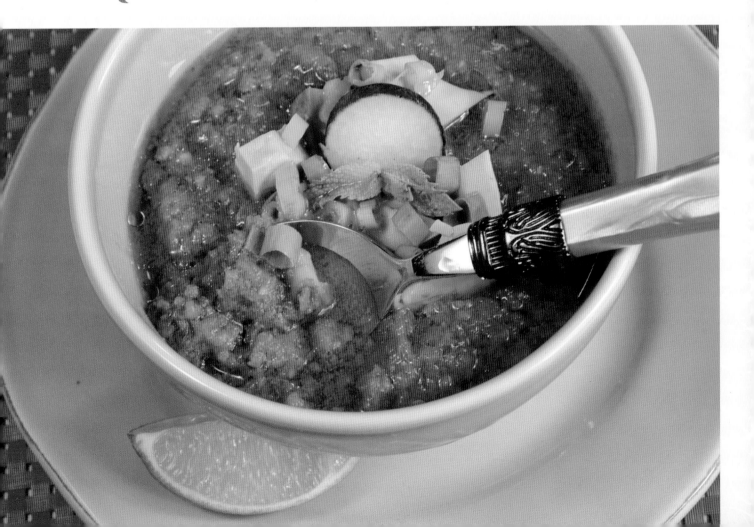

Tapas Salad Picar (a little bite)

2 tomatoes

1 cup arugula

1 sweet red bell pepper

½ sweet red onion

1 large cucumber, English if possible

½ small jalapeño, finely diced (optional)

½ cup green olives

1 avocado, cut into chunks

1 small zucchini

½ cup packed cilantro leaves

Jicama, sliced thinly on mandolin slicer

Dressing

⅛ teaspoon cumin

3 tablespoons good-quality extra-virgin olive oil

Juice from ½ lemon or lime

2 cloves garlic, crushed

Himalayan salt

Freshly milled pepper to taste

DIRECTIONS

Slice jicama thin, but thick enough to have a little body as the salad will be piled on top, like on a tortilla, and eaten by picking up the jicama tortilla. Peel cucumber, and seed tomatoes and peppers. Peel onion, and dice everything into small pieces, except the arugula. Whip the dressing together in a small bowl. Taste for seasonings, and adjust if necessary. Pour on top of chopped salad ingredients, and lightly toss. Chill for 20 minutes, then mound the arugula on top of the jicama, and pile salad on top. The dish is great served on chilled plates with a side slice of lime.

TIP { Mango may also be added to the mix.

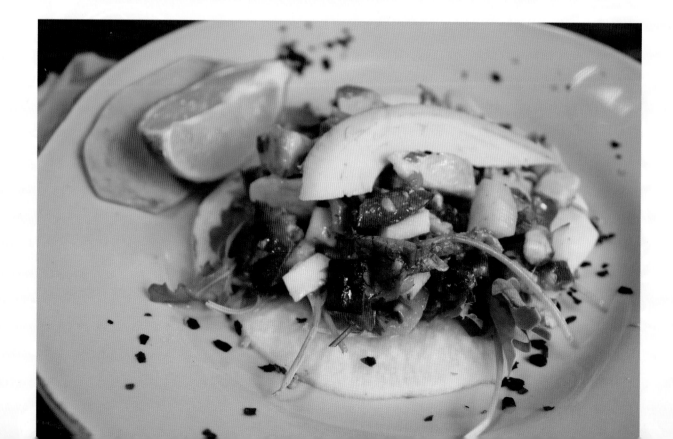

Dinner (La Cena)

SPANISH PIZZA

Although this is an easy recipe, it does take some time to prepare and dehydrate, but don't let that stop you from making this pizza because it's totally satisfying. Pizza crust will freeze very well when wrapped tightly with foil and placed in a Ziploc or airtight bag. This pizza is gluten-free and can be topped with just about anything. Once you master the pizza crust, the toppings are infinite.

Crust

1 cup wet almond pulp

2 cups sprouted buckwheat

2 cups young Thai coconut meat or 1 cup zucchini, peeled

½ cup nutritional yeast, not raw but loaded with B12

3 tablespoons lecithin, nonsoy

½ cup psyllium, ground fine

¼ cup sun-dried tomatoes, soaked until soft

¼ cup of hemp seeds

1 cup flaxseeds, ground to meal

½ small onion, chopped

1 small clove garlic, crushed

1 teaspoon extra-virgin olive oil

Dash of tamari or Bragg's liquid aminos

1 teaspoon lemon juice

1–2 tablespoon Spanish mixed herbs (see p. 52)

Himalayan salt to taste

Freshly milled pepper to taste

Water as needed

DIRECTIONS

In a food processor, blend all ingredients until smooth, except flax meal and psyllium. Scrape down the sides of the processor, and add water if needed to smooth out any lumps. Adjust the salt and herbs to taste. If the crust mixture is not smooth enough, place it in a high-speed blender and blend until smooth. Remove to a bowl, and blend in the flax meal and psyllium by hand. Divide the crust mixture onto 2–3 nonstick dehydrator sheets and shape the dough into large rounds. The crust can also be made into 2 squares. The mixture should be ¾ to 1 inch high. Dehydrate for 4 hours at 110° F, then flip onto a mesh screen and dehydrate for another 8–10 hours or until a light outside crust forms and the inside has a little give.

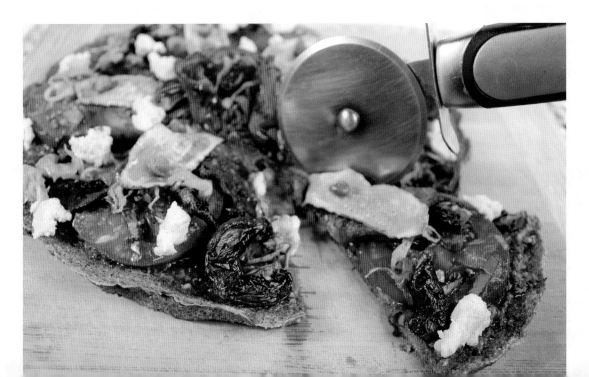

Topping

Use a mandolin slicer or sharp knife to slice red pepper, eggplant, onion, and zucchini thinly.

1 sweet red pepper	12 sun-dried tomato halves, soaked until soft
½ large eggplant	Himalayan salt to taste
1 sweet or red onion	Freshly milled pepper to taste
1 large zucchini	15 olives, cut in half
1 cup crimini mushrooms, sliced thinly	2 tomatoes, thinly sliced
4 tablespoons extra-virgin olive oil	Crumbled nut cheese (see recipe below)
2 tablespoons tamari	Basil pesto (see recipe below)
1 tablespoon Spanish mixed herbs (see p. 52)	¼ cup fresh basil, ribbon cut

DIRECTIONS

Marinate sliced pepper, eggplant, zucchini, mushroom, and onion separately in olive oil, tamari, and Spanish herbs for 15 minutes, turning occasionally. Spread each type of vegetable separately on a nonstick dehydrator tray, and dehydrate for 4 hours at 110° F. They will have a cooked consistency when finished. Slice tomatoes, and marinate in tamari, olive oil, crushed garlic, ribbon-sliced basil, and Spanish herbs.

Pesto

1 cup basil, packed	1 clove garlic
⅛ cup walnuts	Salt to taste
⅛ cup pine nuts	1–2 tablespoons olive oil

DIRECTIONS

Pulse chop walnuts a few times; add basil and garlic and pulse chop until combined. While the processor is running, slowly add 1 tablespoon of the olive oil. Stop to scrape down the sides and check the texture. Add more oil if needed.

Cheese

2 cups macadamia, cashews, or almonds, soaked for 4 hours	2 tablespoons nutritional yeast
1 teaspoon probiotics powder	½ tablespoon lemon juice
½ cup water	Himalayan salt to taste

DIRECTIONS

Drain and place soaked nuts in a blender, adding water as necessary to make a very smooth but thick mixture. Add as much water as needed, a little at a time, to get the mixture moving. Use a tamper to push the mixture down on the sides. Add probiotics. When the mixture is smooth and without lumps, place a strainer lined with cheesecloth or nut filter bag over a bowl, and scrape the cheese mixture into the cloth. Fold up the sides of cheesecloth to cover the top, and place a weight on top. If you used more water to get mixture moving and the cheese is too soft, put some pressure on the weight by gently pushing down with your hand to release some of the liquid, then let the cheese rest with the weight on top on the kitchen counter for 24 hours. Remove the cheese from the cheesecloth, and add nutritional yeast, salt to taste, and lemon juice. Mix well and refrigerate. Leftover cheese can be mixed with pesto or other seasonings and used on raw crackers or bread. It will last 4–5 days in a refrigerator.

Spread pesto on the crust. Spread tomato slices around the crust. Layer on each vegetable one at a time. Crumble on cheese to your liking. Dehydrate to warm or serve at room temperature. Top off with a sprinkle of dried chili peppers for a little kick and with capers if desired. Place on a cutting board, and use a pizza cutter to slice into serving sizes.

Paella (sprouted wild rice with vegetables and spices)

Raw vegan paella might satisfy your taste for this classic local dish. It's a great casual lunch or dinner to share with a group of friends. Creating this dish is like alchemy, turning basic ingredients into a delicious elixir.

Preparation and planning are needed. Chickpeas need sprouting, vegetables need dehydrating, and although paella can be made without dehydrating the vegetable, I think it's worth the time because dehydration gives the dish its complex rich taste. Wild rice must be sprouted overnight, and the final dish, when assembled, must be dehydrated, so plan ahead.

2 cups sprouted wild rice (see p. 44), prepared the night before

1 sweet onion, finely chopped

1–3 cloves garlic, minced

1 sweet red bell pepper, chopped

1 cup eggplant, peeled and chopped

1 large tomato, finely chopped

½ cup sprouted chickpeas, chopped

¾ cup mushrooms, chopped

1 cup zucchini, chopped

1 tablespoon extra-virgin olive oil

Himalayan salt to taste

Freshly milled pepper to taste

2–3 threads of saffron (they are very expensive so can be left out or use ¼ teaspoon saffron powder), soaked in 1 teaspoon water for 20 minutes; use water and threads in recipe

1 teaspoon turmeric

1 teaspoon paprika

½ teaspoon allspice

1 tablespoon Spanish herb mixture (see p. 51)

1 cup peas, freshly shelled, or frozen if fresh not available

1 ear corn, kernels cut from cob

½ cup parsley, leaves only, or spinach leaves, lightly chopped

12 tomatoes that are larger than cherry tomatoes but smaller than plum tomatoes

8 halved sun-dried tomatoes, soaked until soft

¾ cup water

Stock made from juice of 1 carrot, 1 tomato, 1 stalk celery, ¼ cup onion, and 1 clove garlic

8 green olives, cut in half, reserved for garnish

1 tablespoon capers, reserved for garnish

DIRECTIONS

Marinate the chopped onion, red bell pepper, eggplant, mushrooms, and zucchini in tamari and olive oil, turning to absorb liquid for about 10–15 minutes. Spread out on mesh dehydrator screen, and dehydrate at 110° F for 4–5 hours. The vegetables should still be soft, moist, and taste "cooked." Place the rice and remaining ingredients in a mixing bowl, reserving the sun-dried tomatoes and 12 small tomatoes. Mix well and taste for seasonings, adjusting if necessary.

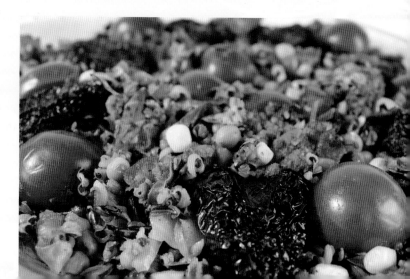

Place the ingredients in large pie pan or glass baking dish, and top around the outside with sliced sun-dried and small tomatoes cut in half and seeded. Dehydrate for 1–2 hours at 115° F or until the top is dry. Cover with foil, and dehydrate overnight or for 9–10 hours. Dehydrate until most or all liquid is gone, which will produce a deep richness to the dish. Add green olives and capers to the finished dish.

TO SERVE

This dish stands on its own with a small, lightly seasoned side salad. A drizzle of good olive oil on top of the paella is also suggested.

Smoked Stuffed Chilies with Creamy Sauce

6 large Anaheim or poblano chilies

1 small sweet onion, finely chopped

4 cloves garlic, crushed

2 serrano chilies, deseeded and finely chopped

1 cup mixed mushrooms, finely chopped

3 medium ripe tomatoes, seeded and cut in quarters

1 cup pecans, chopped

½ cup raisins, soaked to soften

½ teaspoon cinnamon, ground

¼ teaspoon smoked paprika

3 tablespoons fresh oregano, finely chopped, or 1 tablespoon dried

2 teaspoons fresh thyme, finely chopped, or 1 teaspoon dried

Dash of sweetener

Himalayan salt to taste

Freshly milled pepper to taste

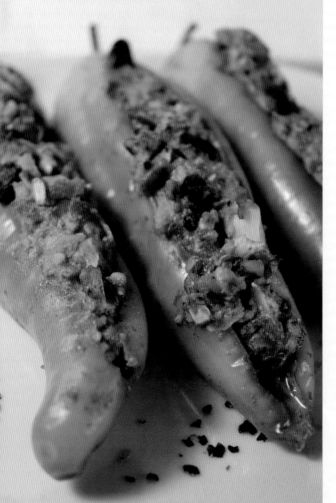

DIRECTIONS

Make a slit in the large chilies, and remove the seeds, keeping the chilies whole for stuffing. Rub with olive oil and half of the smoked paprika, and marinate in a glass baking dish overnight. Turn several times while marinating. Place the remaining ingredients in a bowl, mix well to incorporate, and add in some of the sauce. Stuff the peppers, and place them in the baking dish. Add a little oil and water to the dish, and cover with foil. Place on the bottom shelf of the dehydrator. Dehydrate for approximately 4 hours at 110° F. If using an oven, set at the lowest temperature with the door ajar and watch carefully not to "cook" but just heat peppers.

Creamy Sauce

1 cup cashews, macadamia, or pine nuts

1 cup chopped walnuts

1 Medjool date

¼ teaspoon cacao powder

1–2 cloves garlic

1 teaspoon oregano

1 tablespoon tamari

Freshly milled pepper to taste

Himalayan salt to taste

Water as needed

DIRECTIONS

Blend nuts and water in a high-powered blender until smooth, adding more water if necessary to make a thick, very smooth cream. Scrape down the sides with a spatula. Add the remaining ingredients, and blend. Taste the seasonings, and adjust if necessary.

TO SERVE

To warm the balance of sauce, place in a dehydrator for ½ hour or warm on the stove, taking care to warm to body temperature only. Place a stuffed pepper on a serving plate, and pour sauce on top. Garnish with chopped cilantro or basil.

Dessert (El Postre)

FLAN WITH MAPLE SAUCE (CUSTARD)

½ cup Irish moss gel (see p. 46)

½ cup maple syrup

1 cup young Thai coconut meat

1 cup cashews, soaked for 2 hours

2 teaspoons vanilla extract

½ cup coconut water or pure water, to use as needed

5 tablespoon coconut oil, melted

DIRECTIONS

Grind the nuts in a high-speed blender or spice mill. Remove to a bowl. Add coconut meat, coconut water, and maple syrup in the high-speed blender, then add the nuts back in. Blend until smooth, adding water as needed to keep the mixture moving. The mixture should remain thick but without lumps. Add coconut oil and Irish moss, blending until well incorporated and smooth. Taste for sweeteners, and adjust if necessary. Pour into small molds or flan dishes, and refrigerate until set.

Maple Topping

½ cup maple syrup

TO SERVE

Unmold custard onto a plate, and drizzle 1–2 tablespoons of maple syrup on top. Berries may also be used for topping.

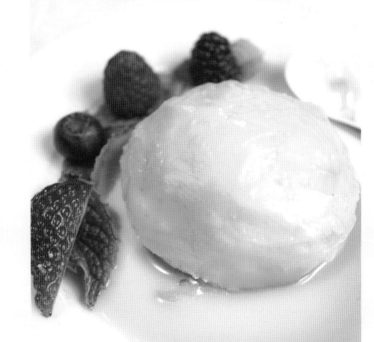

Cinnamon Ice Cream on a Stick

½ teaspoon cinnamon

4 tablespoons maple syrup

Blend together with wire whisk, and set aside.

Ice Cream Base

2½ cups almond milk (see p. 65)

2 cups young Thai coconut meat

2 teaspoons vanilla extract

2 tablespoons coconut oil, melted

4 tablespoons maple syrup or sweetener of choice

DIRECTIONS

Blend all ingredients in a high-speed blender. Taste for sweetness; the mixture should be a bit sweeter than you like, as the sweetness lessens during freezing; add more sweetener if necessary. Add cinnamon to your liking. Once it tastes good to you, pour into a large mason jar with a lid, and refrigerate overnight or for 5 hours. When ready, pour into an ice cream maker, and follow the manufacturer's directions. If you don't have an ice cream maker, place the ice cream into a glass baking dish and freeze. Mix a couple of times to fluff up, or pour into ice cream bar molds. Make a cardboard cover for the mold, and punch a small hole in the center over each ice cream slot. Put a cinnamon stick in each hole for the handle. The cardboard will hold the stick in place until the ice cream is frozen. Tongue depressors can also be used instead of a cinnamon stick and can be purchased at your local pharmacy.

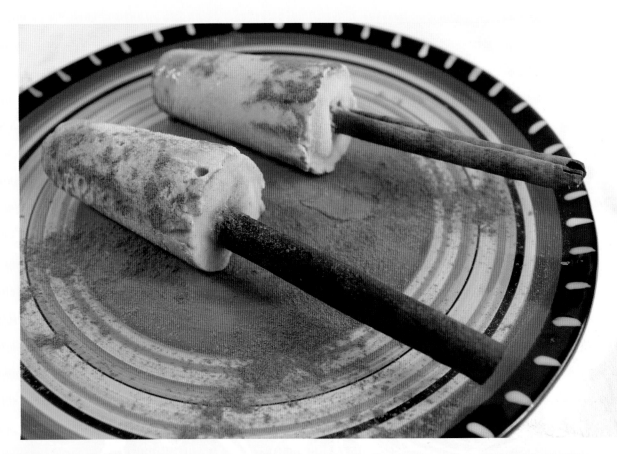

Spiced Dark Chocolate Bark with Hazelnuts

Chocolate can be simple to make once the basics are learned. Chocolate that does not need to be refrigerated after it's hardened is tempered, which means the chocolate is melted, cooled down, then brought up to 88°F a second time. Chocolate that is not tempered is just melted once and placed in a refrigerator or freezer to set. Both can be melted in a double boiler, which is a bowl placed over hot water, also know as a bain-marie, or in Spanish, baño maría. Precautions must be taking when melting cacao butter and coconut oil to prevent water from getting into the batch, which will seize up the mixture. If the mixture seizes add melted cacao butter a little at a time, stirring constantly until smooth. Using the dehydrator method will help with this issue, and it keeps water out of the mixture. It will take a little more time but is much safer. In this recipe I use the dehydrator method and cacao paste instead of cacao powder, which tempers the chocolate on its own.

Chocolate

3¼ cups cacao powder, sifted, or 2½ cups cacao paste, which can be purchased online or in health food stores

1 cup cacao butter

5–6 tablespoons maple syrup or sweetener of choice

1 teaspoon orange extract (see p. 66)

Small pinch of chili powder

1 cup hazelnuts, sliced

Note: Any nuts may be used, but hazelnuts have a sweet taste and contain heart-healthy fats and tons of minerals, including potassium, calcium, magnesium, and vitamins E and B.

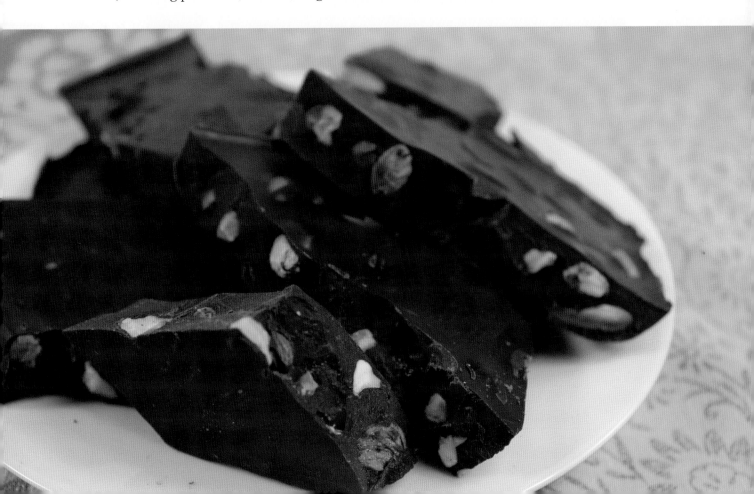

DIRECTIONS FOR NONTEMPERED CHOCOLATE

Melt the cacao butter by placing it in a glass or metal bowl and setting it on top of a pan of boiling water. Stir to break up the pieces. Once the cacao butter is melted, whisk in cacao powder until smooth. Blend in sweetener, extracts, and spice. Place a piece of parchment paper in a glass baking dish, and pour the mixture in, tapping down the dish to distribute the chocolate evenly. Cover the top of the chocolate with sliced hazelnuts. Tap the dish down lightly on the counter to set the nuts in place. Put the dish in a freezer for a quick finish, or place it in a refrigerator to harden. The mixture can also be made in candy molds, but I personally like the bark method for this recipe. The chocolate must be kept refrigerated.

IF YOU ARE USING CACAO PASTE

Melt the cacao butter and paste in a dehydrator or on the stove in a double boiler. Once the lumps start to break up, help along by stirring and encouraging the lumps to melt. When the lumps are almost gone, remove the bowl from the dehydrator, and stir until smooth. Add the remaining ingredients, and blend in. Proceed as above to make chocolate bark. This mixture does not need refrigeration.

Beverages (La Bebida)

SUMMER SANGRIA

2 cups blood orange juice (regular will also work)

2 cups fresh pomegranate or grape juice

½ cup apple juice

½ cup lime juice

1 lemon, thinly sliced, seeds removed

1 orange, thinly sliced, seeds removed

1 apple, cored and thinly sliced

1 peach, thinly sliced, or other fruit in season

Sweetener of choice to taste

2 cups carbonated water, e.g., San Pellegrino

DIRECTIONS

Stir all ingredients except carbonated water in a covered container, and chill overnight in a refrigerator. When ready to serve, place ice in wine glasses, and add ¾ sangria mixture along with some of the fruits. Add sparkling water to fill, and stir. Garnish with mint and a straw. If all the sangria will be consumed in one sitting, add carbonated water directly to the sangria mixture.

 TIP { One carton of raspberries, blended with water and strained of seeds, may be used instead of pomegranate or grape juice.

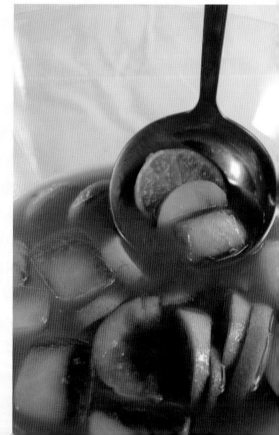

Chocolate Caliente

2 cups almond milk (see p. 65)

3 tablespoons cacao powder or cacao paste

2 tablespoons maple syrup or sweetener of choice

Pinch of cinnamon

Pinch of chili

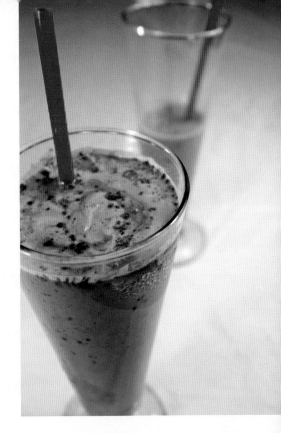

DIRECTIONS

Place all ingredients in a blender, and blend until smooth. If serving cold, add 4–5 ice cubes and blend until cubes disappear. If serving warm, pour into a pan on top of the stove, whisk with wire whisk to make the mixture frothy, and warm to body temperature. Test by sticking a finger in, or use a spoon and drop a bit on the inside of your wrist. Do not overheat. If drinking cold, pour into iced glass with a straw, and garnish with a sprinkling of cinnamon, or if drinking warm, pour into your favorite mug.

Agua Fresca (fresh fruit drink)

Use watermelon, cantaloupe, strawberries, or papaya.

2 cups fresh fruit, coarsely chopped

½ cup sweetener

⅛ cup lime juice

Small amount of water just to achieve desired texture

Pinch of salt

DIRECTIONS

In a high-speed blender add fruit, water, lime juice, and sugar, and blend until smooth. If there are small strawberry seeds in the drink, use a sieve to strain the mixture into a pitcher. Taste for sweetness, and adjust if necessary. Serve well chilled.

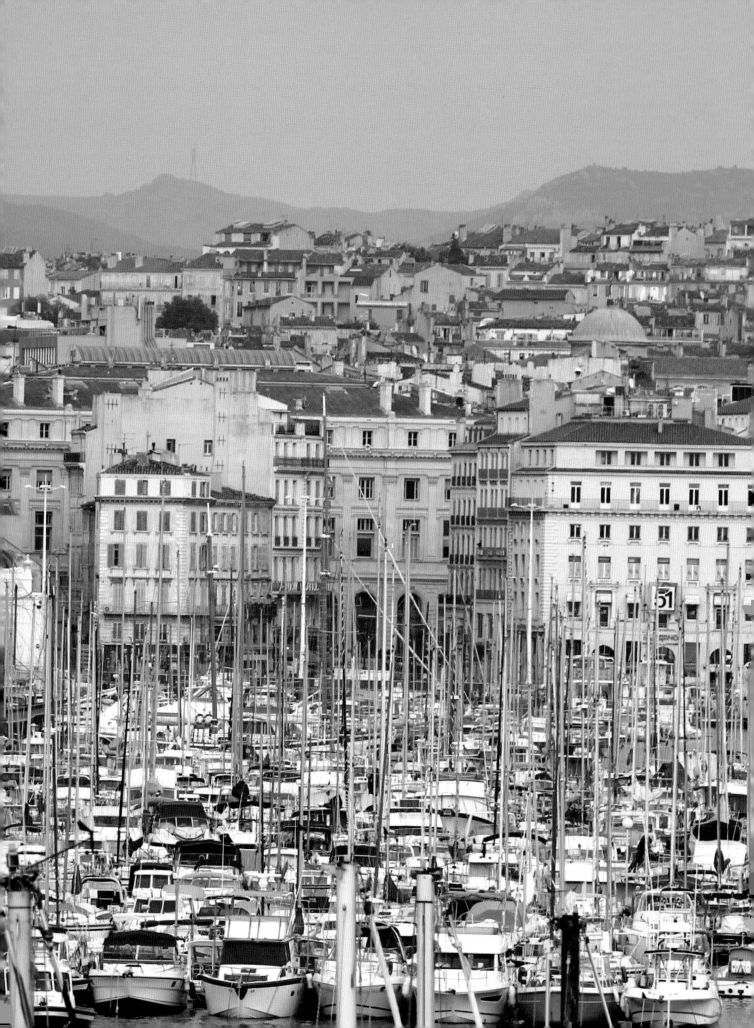

CHAPTER 11

·····················

RAW CUISINE—TASTE OF

FRANCE

·····················

France is the second-largest country in Europe. Its citizens are self-sufficient when it comes to growing their own food. In fact, the French are partial to their way of cooking, so it seems only natural that they prefer their own products over imported ones. Each region and its cultural heritage determines how people eat.

We all know the baguette is a staple in France. I can't say it was easy staying away from this local staple, as everyone seemed to be carrying a loaf or two on his or her way home from the market. Temptation was all around me, but it was a long trip, and gluten is not my friend, so I decided to save my one possible digression for another time.

Each neighborhood has its own character. Little shops carry about everything you need, so you don't have to travel far to find everyday necessities. Our first inclination was to travel to Paris, but after some thought, we changed plans. We've had the pleasure of traveling to Paris and other beautiful cities in France, but on this trip we were drawn to Marseille and Aix-en-Provence because we were still curious about many places we missed when visiting the country previously.

We met up with Windy C. Davis, a friend I met on Facebook. Windy lives in Marseille and showed us around. She even went so far as to contact Chef Kim Jansen at Green Bear, a vegetarian-friendly restaurant, to fix us a raw lunch. Chef Kim, never having prepared raw food before, went online to see what raw food was about and created a tasty cold soup and an extraordinary salad. He later e-mailed me and said he realized he learned to cook in chef school but never learned about nutrition, so now he is extending his talents to learn more about raw food. He is even sprouting now.

Windy took us on a tour of Marseille farmers markets and a spice shop, where the shop owner gave us permission to photograph the spices. Spices were displayed in large burlap bags and beautiful painted tins. I can only tell you that the scent was intoxicating, and the feeling of being in this shop was very exotic. My appreciation for worldly spices grew as I walked around the tiny shop.

Windy also took us to a very old kitchen and hardware store called Maison Empereur, where I purchased a typical pair of Marseille shoes called espadrilles. Espadrilles are rope-bottom shoes with canvas tops, totally vegan, and totally me. We hiked up hills to see spectacular views of Marseille's port and learned some history from Windy.

Tucked in between the hills and the sea, Marseille is the oldest and second-largest city in France and boasts fourteen ports, making it the main sailing center in France. Marseille was founded in 600 BC, and the city continues to modernize itself, but the history is deeply rooted. You can feel its stability, as if everything has always been there and will remain as is. It's a calming feeling to see the new mixed so well with the steadiness of the old. Marseille claims to have 300 days a year of sun and a mild climate. I can assure you, this is a place to paint. The sky is beautiful, and since Marseille is a port city, the water, boats, atmosphere, and lighting can't be matched.

Marseille is a city full of spirit and culture with theaters, outdoor activities, art, music, festivals, and more than seventeen museums to enjoy. Plans for further modernization and exciting changes are in the works to add to this

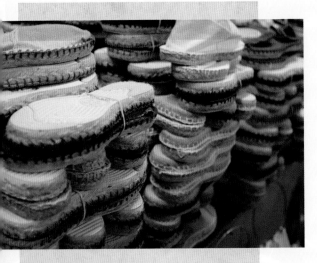

already interesting city. Marseille was chosen to be the Culture Capital of Europe for 2013. The year will be filled with street entertainment, food, photography, open-air concerts, dance, and fireworks. New galleries and venues are open around the city, involving all things cultural.

Marseille is the most filmed city in France next to Paris and occupies an honored place in French cinema. Marseille has a diverse culture with its many immigrant communities from northern Africa and various Mediterranean countries. There is a Moroccan-style souk market with stalls and Moorish ornate shops and restaurants. We checked out Noailles market place, which made my heart pound. Nothing looked familiar. The air was breezy and pungent, and many of the aromas were not familiar to my senses. There is a large North African community with vendors hawking their wares. It's quite exciting, distinctive, and colorful with many men and women in native dress. I was happy to be there.

Marché aux Puces is a premier indoor-outdoor market with uncountable amounts of stalls. You can spend many days looking at food of every nature along with clothing and many ethnic goods. Of course, there are many stalls not fit for vegan eyes. The Prado Market is a daily market that stretches from the Castellane metro station to the Périer metro station with food and wares of every nature, including olive oils, jams, and chocolate. The availability of all this beautiful food only played on me to get into the kitchen and create, but alas, our hotel room did not have one, so I wrote and saved my recipe testing until I arrived back home. We enjoyed plenty of good simple fruits, vegetables, and nuts to keep us happy. It was summer, and the fruits were ripe and juicy. This is how fruit should always taste.

We found many vegetarian-friendly restaurants willing to accommodate my raw preference. When I think of years past when no one even paid attention to requests for vegetarian/vegan food, it's quite exciting to see the growing awareness around the world.

There was a day when I especially felt like a local, not an easy task if you are in a country only for a short time. I was walking through the market shopping for fruits and vegetables, and all of a sudden I had this amazing burst of excitement. The most wonderful feeling rushed over me, and I felt I was living in France. True, it was utterly exciting to be in France writing a chapter for my book, and even though it was not a novel, I felt Hemingway at my side. Could be I saw *Midnight in Paris* one too many times, but Marseille is a romantic city like many in France, and I was swept up in its beauty and history. I looked up from the market street and imagined I lived in one of the apartments in the building above—the one with the scrolled black iron-railed balcony, open double French doors, and sheer curtains moving in the light breeze. Anything can happen when writing a book, even a recipe book. Every thought can be an adventure, and I don't mind absorbing myself in fantasy now and then.

At the markets you can find piles of fruits and vegetables in canopied covered stalls. You can find some organic fare along with prepared salads and other varieties of foods and wines. Every market has its own charm and new foods to discover. The fruit and vegetable stands at each market seemed to look brighter the longer we shopped. I felt there must be nothing left in the farmers' fields as there was such an abundance of foods to choose from every day of the week.

Sun-ripened vegetables, olive oil, and herbs are the basis of many French dishes. Vegetables such as chard, summer squashes, mushrooms, and sweet peppers were abundant. Herbs, including herbes de Provence, nutmeg, mace, rosemary, parsley, oregano, basil, saffron, as well as capers, shallot, and leeks help to create many mouth-watering meals. Our sweet tooth was satisfied with ripe juicy fruits, including melons, peaches, citrus, apricots, cherries, figs, and quince. At a market stall we picked up fresh and delicious pine nuts, almonds, and hazelnuts. They made for great traveling snacks in between meals.

We took a day trip to Aix-en-Provence, pronounced *X en Provence*, hometown of Paul Cézanne, and the city of a thousands fountains. A day is not nearly enough time to spend in this sunny, relaxing town, but we decided to tease ourselves and take a bus to this beautiful gem of a city anyway. Art, music, dance, museums, and plenty of local characters give Aix a special charm and make it one of my favorite towns in the South of France. I could sit in the plaza all day watching the parade of people passing by. Children, dogs, and families all gather to meet and greet every evening. Open-air cafes are full of men and women and the happy sounds wafting out from each place, proving that the French certainly know how to enjoy themselves. A town with therapeutic waters and plenty of spas keeps locals and tourists alike relaxed.

We met up with Marie Tissot, from my Facebook fan page. She lives just outside Aix and brought along a copy of *Live Raw* for me to sign. Her mother was the one who originally told Marie about my book. As we stepped off the bus, there was Marie, a petite, extremely beautiful young woman, who didn't look old enough to be the mother of four. She showed us around Aix, we talked continuously about raw food and life in France. Marie and her husband recently opened a bed-and-breakfast in an old stone house they purchased and are restoring. Mr. Tissot is a winemaker, and they transported their very old grape vines to this new location. If you stay at their B&B, Home Sweet Green, you will find a healthy breakfast including raw, vegetarian, and vegan options. They even have a small apartment with a kitchen you can rent. I fell immediately in love with Marie, and I feel I have a lifelong friend. Find out more about Home Sweet Green at www.facebook.com/HomeSweetGreen.

I like to hunt down restaurants and farmers markets online before leaving home—places where I might find something to eat. Aix, like all French towns, has an abundance of the freshest produce. There is a small everyday market and larger ones that take place once a week. Although people eat salads in abundance, I did not run into anyone who actually knew what raw food was besides Marie, but then again, my French leaves a lot to be desired.

HERBES DE PROVENCE

Herbes de Provence is a beautiful fragrant French mixture I use quite often. It is great in salad dressings, marinades, and soups. For a mixed blend, use a combination consisting of 1 tablespoon each marjoram, tarragon, thyme, chervil, rosemary, and summer savory. Use ½ teaspoon each mint, oregano, and finely chopped bay leaves.

As in many European countries, breakfast consists of coffee, pastries, and breads. After staring into the glass counter at pastry stands, I was delighted not to feel tempted, but it did inspire me to come up with some sweet acceptable French breakfast meals.

Bon Appétit (Enjoy Your Meal)

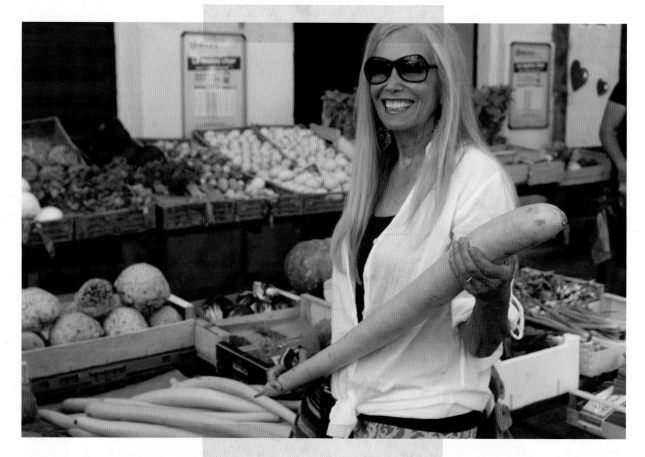

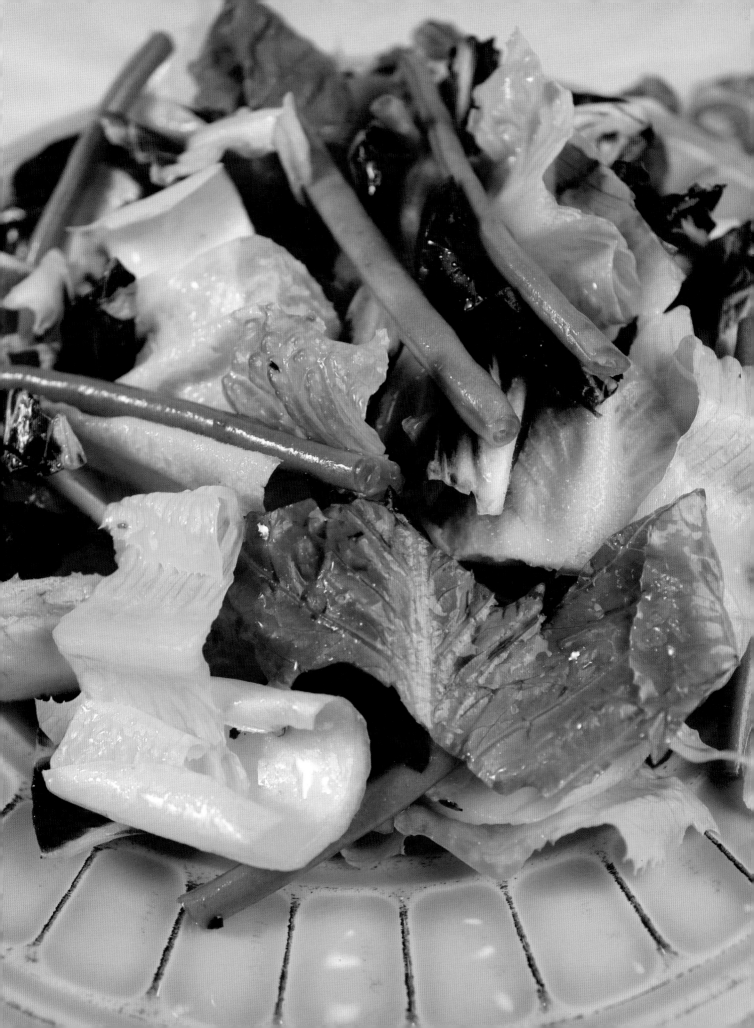

Breakfast (Le Petit Déjeuner)

FRENCH GREEN DRINK WITH SPINACH, PEACH, RASPBERRY, AND LAVENDER

2 peaches or fruit in season	4 Medjool dates
½ carton raspberries	2 drops lavender oil or 2 flowers
2 cups spinach	2 cups water

If you don't have lavender oil to craft this drink into a délicieuse (pronounced *day-lee-seeuhz*) French smoothie, you will need 3 tablespoons fresh lavender flowers or 1½ dried lavender flowers to make a lavender infusion. To make an infusion, boil 2 cups pure water. Place lavender flowers in a teapot or glass container. Let water cool down a bit, then pour water into a teapot or glass container. After 15–20 minutes, strain and use the water for the smoothie. This infusion can be made in the evening and remain refrigerated until ready to use in the morning.

DIRECTIONS
Blend all ingredients in a high-speed blender, including the lavender infusion, until smooth. Ice may be added if desired.

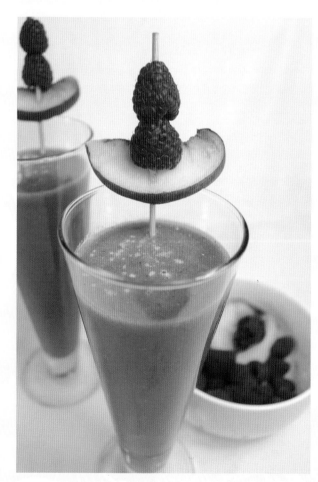

Currant and Cranberry Scone

Although scones are originally from Britain, over time they have become international. Pastry shops all over Europe carry scones, including France, so since the French like sweets for breakfast, I thought this was the right place for these lovely morsels. They have become one of our favorite breakfast treats.

2 cups wet almond pulp

1 cup young Thai coconut meat

½ cup dates, soaked until soft

½ cup flax meal (grind ¼ cup flaxseed to make ½ cup meal)

¼ cup psyllium, ground to fine powder

½ cup buckwheat flour (see p. 44)

⅛ teaspoon cinnamon

½ cup currants or raisins

½ cup cranberries

¾ cups water

DIRECTIONS

Blend coconut meat, dates, and water in a high-speed blender until smooth. In a food processor place almond pulp, flax meal, buckwheat flour, psyllium, and pulse chop until blended. Put all ingredients in a bowl, and add cinnamon, cranberries, and currants, mixing with spatula until everything is well incorporated. Shape into triangles on nonstick dehydrator tray about ½-inch high, and dehydrate for 5–6 hours at 115° F or until desired consistency is reached. Serve warm or at room temperature with cashew cream and fruit jam.

Cashew Cream

1 cup cashews, soaked for 4 hours

2 dates

½ cup young Thai coconut meat (optional but makes cream smoother)

½ teaspoon vanilla extract

½ cup water

DIRECTIONS

Place cashew cream ingredients in a high-speed blender, and process until smooth, adding water to make a thick smooth cream. Add more water if necessary.

Fruit Jam (see pp. 53–54)

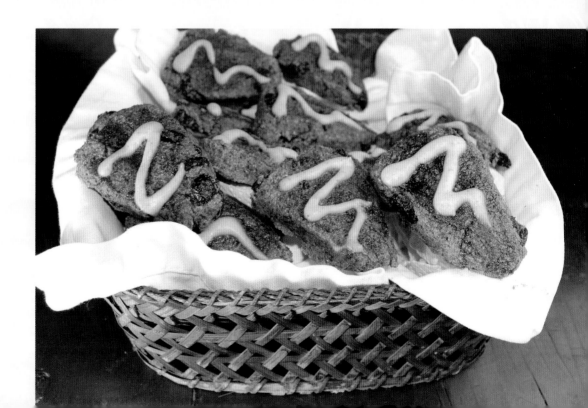

Almond Croissant

3 cups wet almond pulp

2 cups young Thai coconut meat

4 Medjool dates, soaked

½ cup flax meal (grind ¼ cup flaxseed to make ½ cup meal)

¼ cup psyllium

Dash of vanilla

1 teaspoon almond extract

Water as needed

DIRECTIONS

Blend coconut meat and dates until smooth, adding water as needed to make a thick smooth mixture. Scrape into a food processor, and add balance of ingredients. Pulse chop until well combined. The mixture can also be mixed by hand if necessary. The mixture should be thick and moist, but not sticky. Divide it in half, and flatten half on a nonstick dehydrator sheet, making a large square about ¼-inch thick. Use a wet glass to roll smoothly and evenly, wetting the glass as necessary to keep it from sticking. Score through the dough straight down the middle, then side to side, and finally at a diagonal, making 8 triangle shapes. Do the same with the remaining dough. Dehydrate for 3 hours at 110° F until the dough is still pliable. Remove the tray from the dehydrator and separate each piece where it is scored.

Coconut Filling

1 cup dried fine organic coconut (unsweetened)

Beans scraped from one vanilla stick or 1 teaspoon vanilla extract

⅔ cup maple syrup or sweetener of choice

½ teaspoon almond extract

6 tablespoons coconut butter (this is different from coconut oil; I use Artisana)

DIRECTIONS

Place all ingredients in a bowl, and mix together well. Place the mixture in a refrigerator to harden for 15–20 minutes for perfect texture.

TO ASSEMBLE

Place a small amount of filling in the center, and with the pointed end closest to you, fold over the pointed end away from you over the wide end. Bring the sides around towards you, pinching the dough and ends and making a crescent shape. The dough is very pliable, so you can shape the croissant easily. Place back in the dehydrator when all croissants are filled and shaped. Dehydrate for another 3–4 hours at 110° F. The final product will be slightly soft. It is best served warm.

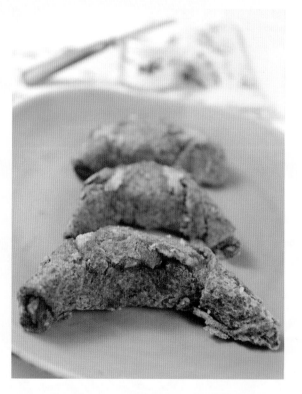

Rustic Artesian Noir Bread with Raisin, Walnut, and Cinnamon

Chef Ito, one of my favorite chefs from Au Lac Restaurant in Southern California, inspired me to make bread recipes.

Makes 2 loaves:

2 cups wet almond pulp

2 cups young coconut meat

1 cup psyllium, ground finely

½ cup flax meal (grind ¼ cup flaxseed to make ½ cup meal)

3 teaspoons lemon juice

6 Medjool dates, soaked until soft

2 teaspoons cinnamon

1 cup walnuts, chopped

1 cup raisins, soaked in 1½ cups water; reserve soaking water

½ banana, mashed

Dash of Himalayan salt

DIRECTIONS

Place coconut meat, dates, and ½ cup raisin soaking water in a high-speed blender. Add more water if needed to blend the mixture until smooth. In a food processor place coconut mixture, almond pulp, psyllium meal, flax meal, lemon juice, cinnamon, and pulse chop until well incorporated. Place all ingredients into a bowl, and add, walnuts, raisins, and mashed banana. Blend well with a spatula or use hands if necessary. Add more raisin water if necessary to achieve smooth, pliable dough. Taste dough, and add more cinnamon and maple syrup if necessary. Bread should have a sweet taste and enough cinnamon to your liking. Divide the mixture in half, and pack each loaf firmly between your hands, making 2 small, oval-shaped loaves. Place both loaves on a mesh dehydrator sheet. Brush the tops with a mixture of cinnamon and maple syrup. Set the dehydrator on 115° F, and dehydrate for 12–14 hours. Eat with jam or sweet cheese.

Cheese Spread—Sweet or Savory

1 cup cashews

½ cup water

½ teaspoon probiotic powder for fermenting

1 teaspoon lemon juice

½ cup Irish moss gel (see p. 46)

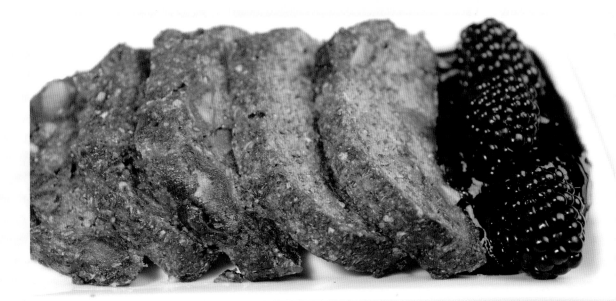

Blend all ingredients in a high-speed blender until smooth and thick, adding water if necessary. Line a strainer with a piece of cheesecloth, and scoop the cheese into the cloth. Bring up the ends to cover the cheese. Put a plate with a weight on top to extract the liquid. Allow cheese to sit in a warm spot in your kitchen for 24 hours. Undo the cheesecloth, add Irish moss, and mix well. Add maple syrup or a sweetener of choice for a sweet cheese, or herbs of choice for a more savory taste. Herbes de Provence work very well with this cheese. Add a pinch of Himalayan salt if necessary. Refrigerate the cheese. The cheese can be made in advance and stored for a few days. Expect a cream cheese texture.

TO SERVE

When ready to serve, cut the bread in ¼-inch or so rounds the short way. Place the bread, cheese, and jam on a plate. The bread is also good warmed in a dehydrator before serving if preferred.

For the jam or marmalade, see pp. 53-55.

Lunch (Le Déjeuner)

Lunch in France is so wonderful. Everything stops for lunch. Stores close between twelve and two, and in summer sometimes they stay closed until four. How civilized! Many of us would love to adopt the long, leisurely lunches the Europeans enjoy, but alas, we are always in a hurry. Many Americans choose fast food restaurants for their lunchtime meal, and in less than one hour they are back at their jobs long before their food has had time to be digested. It's enjoyable to take a break in the middle of the day and sit at a sidewalk café watching people *les bisous* (air-kissing on either side of the face), but it's healthy for both mind and body to relax while eating. Taking time to meet with friends and enjoy a meal can only encourage a better outlook on life. It feels like such a luxury to dawdle when it should feel natural.

A good-sized meal at lunch is a good thing as long as you enjoy a smaller dinner. So many of us don't have time for a long leisurely lunch, so we tend to eat a smaller fast lunch and rush right through it. Do your best to savor the little time you might have by chewing slowly and taking a few deep breaths here and there. Remember to make the best food choices you can, whatever the circumstance.

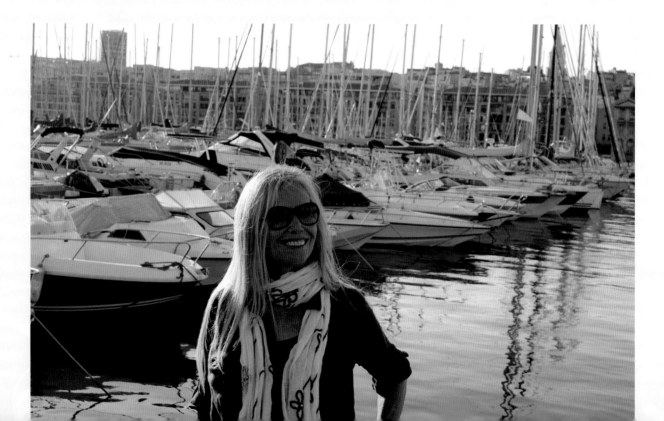

Endive, Haricot Verts Salad with Tarragon Vinaigrette

Haricot vert is a French green bean, which is long, tender, and very dark green. If you can't find it at your market, use a thin green bean. Serving this salad on chilled plates adds a touch of French class. Place the salad plates in a freezer for 1–2 hours before serving.

Note: The evening before you make this salad, marinate 2 fresh stems tarragon, or 1 teaspoon dried, in ⅛ cup apple cider vinegar. Just place the tarragon in vinegar before starting the basic recipe if short on time.

3 Belgian endives (remove leaves one at a time; cut away core as you go; cut leaves in chunks)

20 haricot verts or string beans, ends cut

1 head radicchio or red lettuce, cored and broken in pieces

1 head romaine lettuce, broken in pieces

4 leaves butter lettuce

Wash and spin dry all lettuce

DIRECTIONS

Using a wire whisk, mix together. Toss all ingredients in a bowl except the butter lettuce.

Dressing

1 clove pressed garlic

¼ teaspoon Dijon or homemade mustard (see p. 54)

Small dash of maple syrup or sweetener of choice

Himalayan salt to taste

Freshly ground pepper to taste

⅛ cup apple cider vinegar marinated with 1 stem of tarragon

½ cup good-quality organic cold-pressed olive oil

DIRECTIONS

Taste the dressing, and adjust the seasonings if necessary. Toss with the salad ingredients, reserving the butter lettuce. Place the butter lettuce on a chilled plate, and pile the mixed salad on top.

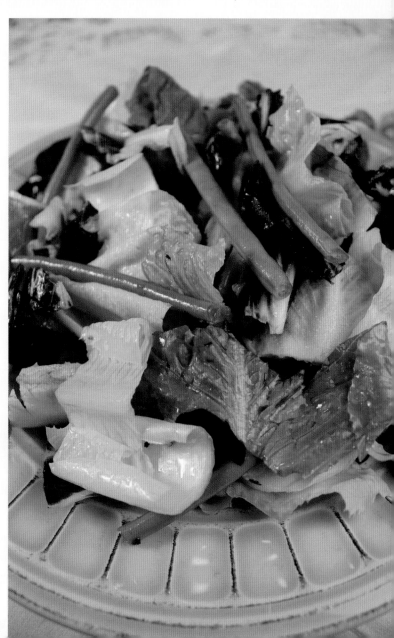

Tomato, Zucchini, Caramelized Onion Tart

2 individual tart pans with removable bottoms

Tart Crust

1½ cups cashews

2 tablespoons flaxseed, ground to meal

1 clove garlic, crushed

¼ cup zucchini, coarsely chopped

¼ cup black olives, raw if possible

1 tablespoon basil, chopped

1 teaspoon thyme

1 tablespoon nutritional yeast

1 teaspoon extra-virgin olive oil

1 teaspoon lemon juice

Pinch of salt

1 tablespoon water or more, if needed, to help crust stick together

DIRECTIONS

Place all ingredients in a food processor, and grind until smooth. Press into tart pans with a removable bottom, and place in a dehydrator for 5–6 hours at 115° F.

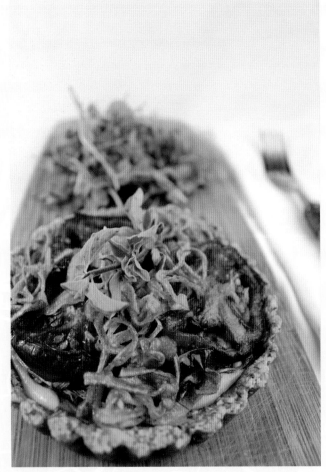

Vegetable Filling

2 tomatoes, thinly sliced

1 large zucchini, thinly sliced on mandolin slicer if possible

DIRECTIONS

Marinate the tomatoes and zucchini in oil and tamari for 15 minutes. Place the slices on a nonstick dehydrator sheet, and dehydrate for 3 hours at 110° F until softened.

Caramelized Topping

3 large onions, thinly sliced with mandolin slicer if possible

4 Medjool dates, soaked

Dash of tamari

2 tablespoons extra-virgin olive oil

2–3 tablespoons water

Himalayan salt to taste

DIRECTIONS

Blend dates, tamari, olive oil, water, and salt until smooth. Place thinly sliced onions in a bowl and pour marinade over top. Mix until onions are completely covered. Dehydrate on nonstick dehydrator sheet for 3 hours at 110° F.

Cheese Filling

1 cup cashews, soaked for 3 hours	2 tablespoons nutritional yeast
1 zucchini	Himalayan salt to taste
¼ cup water, or more if needed	Freshly milled pepper to taste
1 tablespoon organic unpasteurized miso	

DIRECTIONS

Place all ingredients in a high-speed blender except water. Use half of the water to start, and slowly add when needed to make a thick but smooth mixture. Taste for salt and pepper, and adjust if necessary.

TO ASSEMBLE

Place a layer of sauce on the crust, followed by softened zucchini. Sprinkle half of the caramelized onions on top. Place a layer of sliced tomatoes on top, and finish with a balance of onions. Place in a dehydrator until the cheese forms a crust and settles in the tart.

SERVING

Serve with a simple green salad.

Wilted Spinach Apple Salad with Warm Shallot Vinaigrette

4 cups spinach	½ cup raisins
2 apples, thinly sliced	½ cup walnuts, broken in pieces

Vinaigrette

½ cup cold-pressed extra-virgin olive oil	¼ teaspoon Dijon or homemade mustard (p. 54)
1–2 shallots, finely chopped	Pinch of Himalayan salt
2 tablespoons lemon juice	Freshly ground pepper to taste

DIRECTIONS

In a large salad bowl, place spinach, apple, raisins, and walnuts. Place all dressing ingredients in a small bowl, and briskly whisk until well incorporated. Warm the dressing until it reaches body temperature, but be careful to not overheat. Pour the dressing over the salad, and gently toss to coat the salad. Mill freshly ground pepper on top.

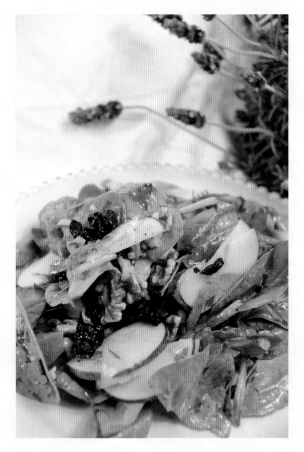

Dinner (Le Dîner)

Vegetable Brochette with Assorted Sauces

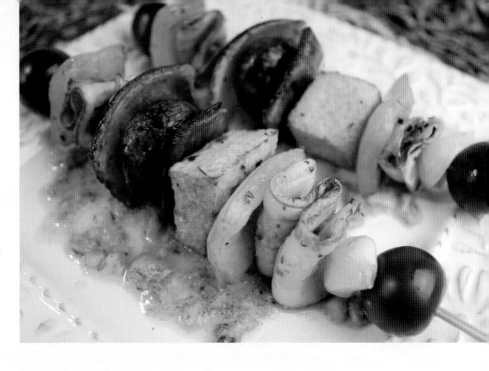

Fresh, colorful, and light vegetable brochettes are satisfying and quick. They make a beautiful presentation on their wooden skewers, and the sauces can range from mild to spicy to exotic.

For 6 skewers use:

- 2 zucchinis, sliced lengthwise (on mandolin slicer or with potato peeler) into 12 slices
- 12 cherry tomatoes
- 1 red bell pepper, cut into 1-inch square pieces, 12 total
- 1 yellow bell pepper, cut into 1-inch square pieces, 12 total

- 1 jicama, cut into small cubes and marinated, 12 total
- 1 very sweet red onion, cut in half, peeled and cut into 1-inch pieces, 12 total
- 6 marinated cloves garlic (optional; see recipe below)
- 6 button mushrooms, destemmed and wiped clean with damp paper towel

DIRECTIONS

Vegetable Marinade

- 2 tablespoons olive oil
- 2 tablespoons gluten-free tamari
- 2 cloves garlic, crushed

- 1 teaspoon herbes de Provence
- 1 tablespoon sweet or spicy paprika

DIRECTIONS

Whisk the marinade ingredients together, and toss in the vegetables. Marinate for 1 or more hours. Place the vegetables on the mesh screen of a dehydrator tray. Dehydrate for 2½–3 hours at 115° F, which will give the vegetables a cooked taste and texture. When the veggies are ready, thread them onto wooden skewers alternating cherry tomato, garlic, zucchini slices (ribbon up), yellow bell pepper, jicama, red bell pepper, mushroom, and onion. Repeat, leaving off the tomatoes and garlic, and end each skewer with a tomato.

Garlic Marinade

Even if you don't use garlic cloves for this recipe, it's nice to keep in your refrigerator. The oil and cloves can be used for salads and other dishes. This is also a nice gift to bring to someone's home.

2 garlic bulbs

½ cup olive oil or enough to cover

½ teaspoon peppercorns

1 tablespoon fresh thyme leaves

¼ teaspoon onion seeds or chopped shallots

1 teaspoon dried basil

DIRECTIONS

Separate and peel the garlic cloves. Place all ingredients in a small mason jar and cover. Store in a refrigerator for 5–7 days.

The French Love Their Sauces

SAUCE 1

1½ teaspoons Dijon or other French mustard or homemade mustard (see p. 54)

1 tablespoon capers, crushed in garlic press

1 clove garlic, crushed

½ teaspoon tarragon

8 tablespoons olive oil

½ cup pine nuts

Freshly milled pepper to taste

Himalayan salt to taste

DIRECTIONS

Place all ingredients in a high-speed blender, and process until very smooth, adding water drop by drop until desired consistency is reached.

SAUCE 2

½ cup olive oil

2 tablespoons lemon juice

2 tablespoons tamari

¼ cup shallots, finely chopped

2 cloves garlic, crushed

½ teaspoon Dijon or homemade mustard (see p. 54)

⅛ teaspoon herbes de Provence

Whisk all ingredients in a bowl, and let marinate for 3–4 hours or more. Can be spooned over skewers when ready to serve.

TO SERVE

Place 6 skewered brochettes on a platter. Put dipping sauce in 2 small bowls with spoons for serving, and place them next to the brochette platter.

TIPS { Other light dipping sauces can be made more spicy or sweet.

Portobello Steak au Poivre

Steak au Poivre is a very popular French dish. We are switching out the steak for portobello mushrooms. The au poivre sauce and the encrusted pepper are what make this dish stand out.

2 large portobello mushroom caps

DIRECTIONS

Wipe the top of the mushrooms with a damp paper towel. Turn the mushrooms over, and with a butter knife or teaspoon, carefully remove the dark gills. When finished removing the gills, use a long serrated bread knife and, holding the round part of the mushroom in your palm, slice off the thin edge around the mushroom that curls in towards the center. This leaves a nice solid mushroom steak. Pat the mushrooms dry with a paper towel, and place in marinade. Marinate for 1 hour, turning the mushrooms a few times to absorb the marinade.

Marinade for Mushrooms

1 large clove garlic, crushed	2 tablespoons olive oil
2 tablespoons tamari	1 tablespoon water
1 tablespoon umeboshi paste	Water as needed

DIRECTIONS

Grind a good amount of semicourse black pepper and press onto round side of mushroom with back of a tablespoon. Dehydrate round side down on mesh screen for 1½–2 hours at 110°F. When mushrooms are ready, slice each cap at an angle and fan on plate.

Au Poivre Sauce

2 tablespoons olive oil	2 teaspoons cognac or brandy (optional but makes the taste authentic and quite yummy)
1½ tablespoons shallots, finely chopped	
Pinch of salt	4 tablespoons almond milk

DIRECTIONS

Pour the olive oil in a small frying pan, and heat it to body temperature. Place the shallots in the pan, stir, and let warm for a minute. Shut the flame off so as not to overheat the mixture, and let it cool slightly on the burner. Turn the flame back on, and warm again. Shut the flame off, and add the cognac or brandy. Light the liquid in the pan with a long torch lighter (used for barbecue or candle lighting) or a long barbecue match. Don't use a regular short match, as the flames in the pan come jumping up immediately and could burn you. Pick up the handle of the pan and shake it while the flames are going. The flames will subside in a few seconds. Place the pan back on the stove, and add almond milk. Mix well, and warm a bit. Pour on top of the sliced mushrooms.

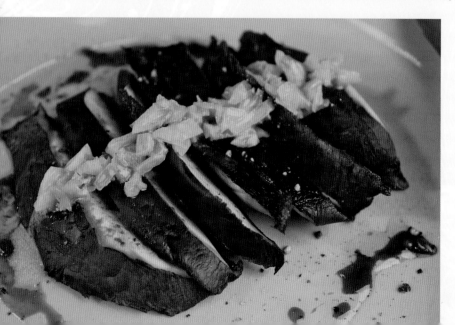

Veggie Bouillabaisse

Bouillabaisse is originally a fish stew originating from the port city of Marseille. Not to insult the French, but I knew I could make a decent raw veggie version by using seaweeds to accomplish a seaworthy taste.

PART 1: STOCK

¼ cup shallots, finely chopped

2 celery ribs, finely chopped

½ fennel bulb, finely chopped

1 leek, white part only, finely chopped

3 cloves garlic, chopped

1 strip orange zest

2 tomatoes, seeded and finely chopped

DIRECTIONS

Marinate all vegetables for 15 minutes in tamari, olive oil, and a little water. Place on the mesh screen of a dehydrator tray, and dehydrate for 2½ hours until softened. When finished, place the vegetables in a glass bowl and add:

¼ cup parsley, leaves only

¼ teaspoon turmeric

2 pistils of saffron or ½ teaspoon saffron powder

¼ cup kombu seaweed, soaked till soft

¼ cup hijiki seaweed, soaked till soft

1 teaspoon dulce flakes

1 heaping teaspoon herbes de Provence

3 cups water

Himalayan sea salt to taste (½ teaspoon or more)

Freshly milled pepper to taste

Small pinch cayenne pepper

Dash of tamari

PART 2: VEGETABLES

½ medium eggplant, peeled, deseeded, and chopped

1 carrot, chopped

1 zucchini, chopped

½ cup mushrooms, wiped clean and cut in small pieces (use shiitaki, cremini or portobello)

1 yellow or red sweet pepper, chopped

Marinade

2 tablespoons tamari

3 tablespoons extra-virgin olive oil

1 tablespoon water

1 tablespoon herbes de Provence

DIRECTIONS

Marinate the chopped vegetables, turning and mixing 3–4 times for 1 hour. Spread all vegetables onto the mesh screen of a dehydrator, and dehydrate for 2–3 hours until they are softened.

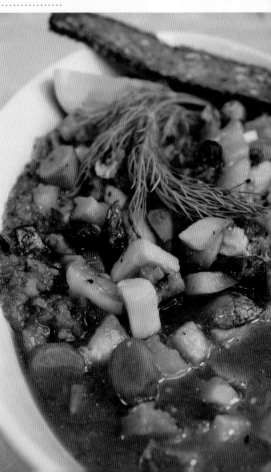

Place the dehydrated stock vegetables (part 1) in a blender, and blend until semismooth, leaving a little texture. Place them in a large mixing bowl. Add the dehydrated marinated vegetables (part 2), and mix together. Taste for salt, pepper, and other spices, and add more if necessary.

TO SERVE

Warm on the stove or in a dehydrator to body temperature. Ladle into soup bowls, and serve a side of crushed chili pepper for those who like a little spice.

Dessert (Le Dessert)

French Lemon Custard

1 cup lemon juice

½ avocado

⅓ cup Irish moss (see p. 46)

5 tablespoons water

⅛ teaspoon turmeric, for color

½–¾ cup maple syrup or sweetener of choice

7 tablespoons coconut oil

DIRECTIONS

Place all ingredients except coconut oil and half of the water in a high-speed blender, and blend until smooth. Add coconut oil, and by the spoonful add a balance of water until a smooth texture is achieved. Blend until well incorporated. Place in ramekins, or cut lemons lengthwise and scoop out center. Fill the cavities with lemon mixture, and refrigerate or freeze until set.

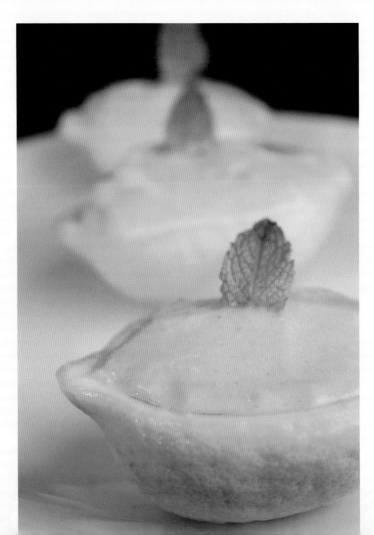

Lavender Ice Cream

3 cups almond or cashew milk (see p. 65)

2–3 tablespoons organic culinary lavender flowers or ½ teaspoon lavender oil (see p. 98)

2 tablespoons coconut oil

⅓ cup liquid sweetener of choice

1 vanilla bean, seeds scraped from inside, or 1 teaspoon vanilla extract

Meat of young Thai coconut (optional)

DIRECTIONS

Place all ingredients except lavender in a high-speed blender, and blend until smooth. Taste for sweetness, and add more sweetener if necessary. Add lavender a drop at a time, tasting as you go. The mixture should taste a little sweeter than you want, as freezing changes the sweetness. Pour the mixture into a container with a lid, and place in a refrigerator overnight or for at least 4 hours. When ready, pour into an ice cream maker and follow the manufacturer's direction. If you don't have an ice cream maker, place in a freezer to set. Take out 10 minutes before serving, and as soon as it slightly softens, mix well with a fork to fluff up.

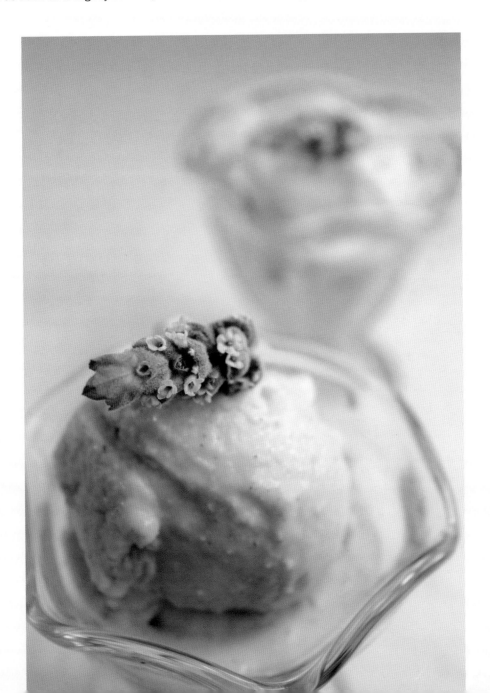

Raspberry Crème Brûlée

1 carton raspberries plus some for topping	5 generous tablespoons Irish moss (see p. 46)
½ cup cashews	Pinch of salt
½ cup macadamia nuts	2 teaspoons vanilla extract
4 tablespoons coconut oil, melted	Water as needed (add 1 tablespoon at a time)
6 tablespoons maple syrup or sweetener of choice	

Topping

Maple syrup, coconut nectar, or agave

DIRECTIONS

Grind the cashews in a high-powered blender or spice mill to make powder. Grind the macadamia nuts into powder in the same manner. Add all ingredients to a blender, and blend until very smooth, using a tamper and only adding enough water to get the mix moving. Keep it thick. Taste for sweetness to your liking.

TO SERVE

Spoon the mixture into ramekins, flatten the top, and tap down. Unmold after chilling for 4 hours or overnight. Pour the topping on, and add fresh raspberries.

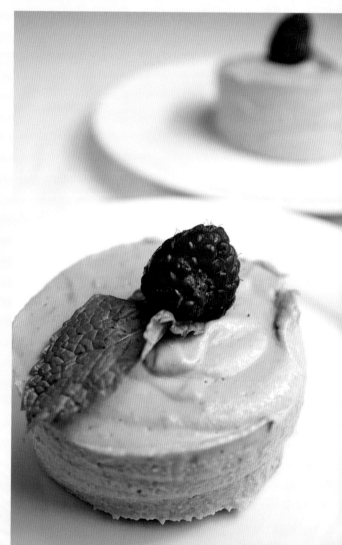

Drinks (Les Boissons)

Limeade Frosty

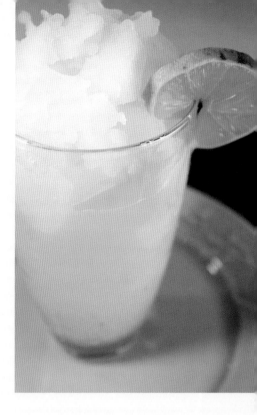

1 cup lime juice

1 tablespoon lime zest

Sweetener of choice to taste

Dash of lemon verbena extract (see p. 66) or fresh mint

1 cup ice

San Pellegrino or other sparkling water

DIRECTIONS

Place all ingredients except the sparkling water in a high-speed blender. Blend until smooth and thick. Taste for sweetness, and adjust if necessary. Pour into long-stemmed glasses, add sparkling water, and stir. Garnish with lime zest and a sprig of mint.

TIP { Before filling the glasses, wet the rims with a little limeade, and dip in coconut sugar.

Lavender Mint Tea

1–2 stems of fresh mint

3 teaspoons dried culinary lavender flowers (unsprayed) or 1–2 drops lavender oil (see p. 98)

Sweetener of choice to taste

DIRECTIONS

Place the mint, lavender, and sweetener in a mason jar filled with water. Place the jar in the sun to make sun tea. Warm to body temperature in a pan. The water can also be boiled and cooled down, and the mint, lavender, and sweetener can be added then.

TIP { Add chamomile, rosemary, or fennel for a variety of taste.

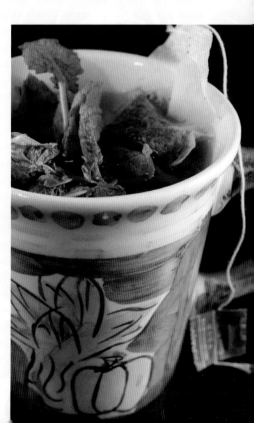

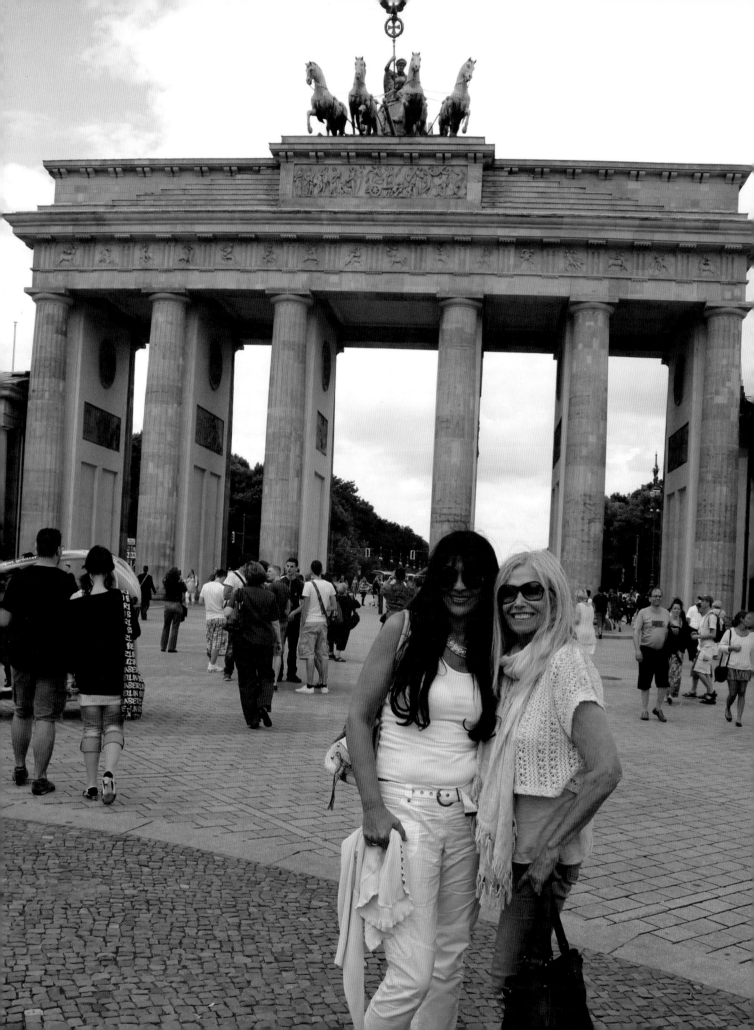

CHAPTER 13

....

RAW CUISINE—TASTE OF

GERMANY

....

When I decided to include German recipes, we took quite a while to decide which city to visit. Since my first recipe book, *Live Raw*, was published in German, I have many social-media friends all around Germany. We ended up choosing Berlin for several reasons. One reason was the history of the Berlin Wall, the modern architecture, and the many friends I had made contact with online.

We were greeted in our hotel room by a beautiful bouquet of pink roses sent by Dorte, a Facebook friend, who took us on a tour of her city. We hit it off immediately, just like old girlfriends who hadn't seen each other for a while. I've always wanted to see the Berlin Wall, but, of course, there is only a small piece standing where it once separated east and west. It's hard to believe the wall went up overnight, leaving families separated for 30 years. You get the sense that although Berlin is still rebuilding, the citizens do not want to erase their history. Our tour took us through old and new Berlin, and the feeling we had was both sad for the past during Hitler's regime and the Cold War years afterward and happy to see the rebuilding of a beautiful city with loving people.

Another new friend we met up with is a talented singer who goes by the name of Karla Stereochemistry. We were lucky enough to see one of her club performances and the following day met up with her for lunch in a local historical neighborhood. We had a simple meal and learned more of Berlin's history of neighborhoods that had been completely bombed out and then rebuilt.

I had been corresponding online with Nick Eii, a Romanian man who was spending a short time in Berlin. He invited us to a beautiful yoga school/ashram to meet his friends, see their green yard and small organic shop, and have lunch. He thoughtfully had the cook fix us a raw meal, and we were surprised to find that she had never prepared one before. The ashram is already health-minded, but after our meeting they planned on including more raw food on their menu. They quickly realized how beneficial raw food is for health and overall well-being. The ashram is a beautiful peaceful place, where rooms are rented to those coming to visit and practice yoga. We sat in the garden with a small group and spoke of many common experiences in our lives and spiritual paths. One of the wonderful things about traveling is meeting like-minded people from other parts of the world and sharing common thoughts about love and peace around the globe.

There was so much to see and learn about Berlin, but as you might have guessed by now, I'm a sucker for farmers markets, which are the mainstay for daily household shopping in most European countries. We found a Turkish market with mounds of dried fruits, nuts, and spices. The aroma of nutmeg and cinnamon came wafting up my nostrils, and I was lost, not knowing what country I was in for a moment. There was a different market to go to every day, and each had its own charm.

I also love flea markets for their culture and special finds. We went to so many flea markets on our trip that in Berlin, Mike gave me a roll of the eyes to let me know we were finished shopping and that our suitcases were full.

Berlin has many vegetarian and vegan restaurants. I gave a talk one evening at one of the best vegan and raw restaurants I've ever enjoyed. La Mano Verde opened up five years ago and was voted in the top 800 restaurants of all Europe. It serves both raw and vegan dishes. The owner, Jean Jury, a very charming Frenchman who is passionate about good food, sat us in the patio for dinner after my talk. We were served course after course; each one was more beautiful to look at than the last, and each course was amazingly delicious. Mike and I finished every bite, and I was in raw food heaven. Jean and I share the importance of starting with the best and freshest ingredients you can buy, and he is devoted to bringing the best quality and extraordinarily tasty food to the table of his clientele. Jean is a fellow foodie, and I just fell in love with this man and what he is doing for the growth of raw and vegan food popularity. Once people taste his dishes, they will completely understand how good raw food can be even if they normally consume a standard diet. I think the most discerning gourmet would agree that eating at La Mano Verde could convince them to include more raw foods in his or her diet.

We also had the pleasure of dining at one of Chef Boris Lauser's dinner parties. Boris is a thin, muscular, healthy-looking young raw food chef. He holds occasional raw food dinner parties in his flat. They're not to be missed if you ever travel to Berlin. He is a lovely host, and he prepares many raw food courses at his parties. Boris was trained at the Matthew Kenny Academy and is a star on the raw food scene throughout Germany and beyond. He is a guest chef and gives classes at La Mano Verde.

My addiction and challenge of new ways to fix raw German food continues. What is German food, you ask, without potatoes, sauerkraut, and sausage? I wondered the same thing, but once I understood what herbs and spices are used, I was on a mission. Here is a surprising fact you might not know: There are over 30,000 vegetarian, vegan, and raw foodists throughout Germany, and their numbers are steadily growing.

german herbs and spices

German food is not spicy. In fact, I consider it very mild tasting. Spices such as parsley root, marjoram, caraway, chives, dill weed, anise, borage, lovage, and paprika are a few of those that German cooks favor. You may also find thyme, laurel, and more recently basil, sage, and oregano in many dishes.

When it comes to condiments, mustard is at the top of the list. Mustard can be sweet, medium, hot, or grainy. You will find mustard on every table. Horseradish is another condiment that honors German food. There are many outside influences today playing a part in German traditional food, including Italian, French, Spanish, Greek, and Portuguese.

Just like we have our pumpkin pie spice, Germany has its own spice mixture called Lebkuchen. It's similar to ours except for the addition of anise. This mixture can be used in many desserts and even in warm almond milk to make a lovely breakfast drink. (See p. 52 for savory German spices.)

lebkuchen (spice mixture)

2 tablespoons cinnamon

2 teaspoons cloves

½ teaspoon allspice

¼ teaspoon nutmeg

½ teaspoon each cardamom, coriander, ginger, and anise seeds

DIRECTIONS

All spices should be ground. Mix them together, and place the mixture in an airtight container. Store in a dark, dry place.

Guten Appetit (Enjoy Your Meal)

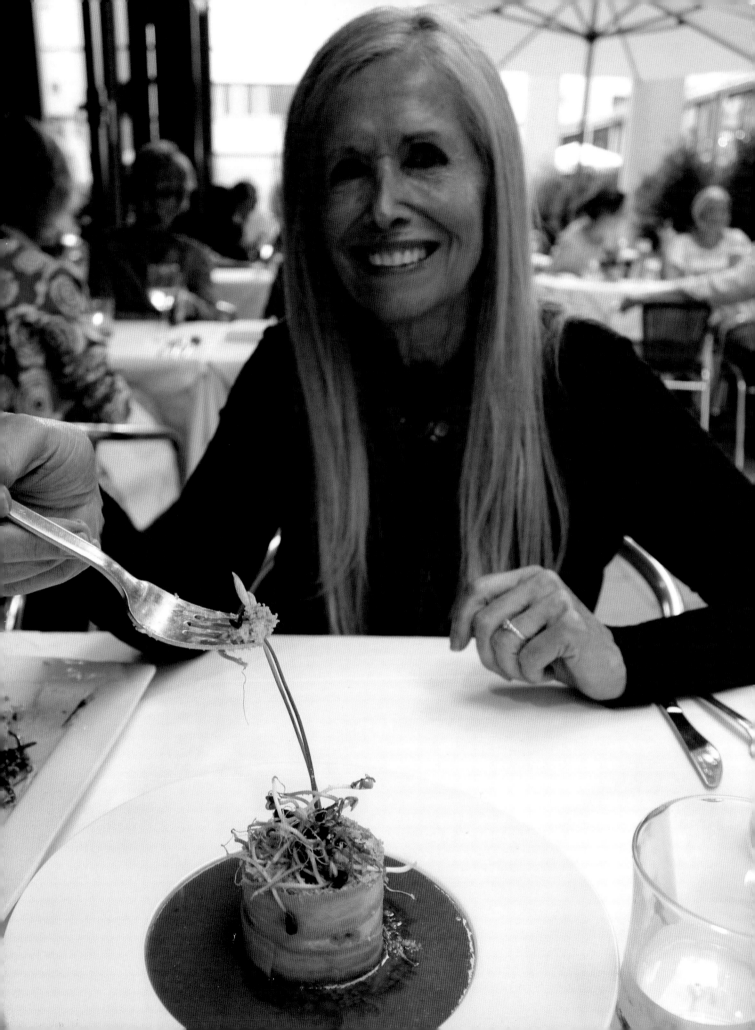

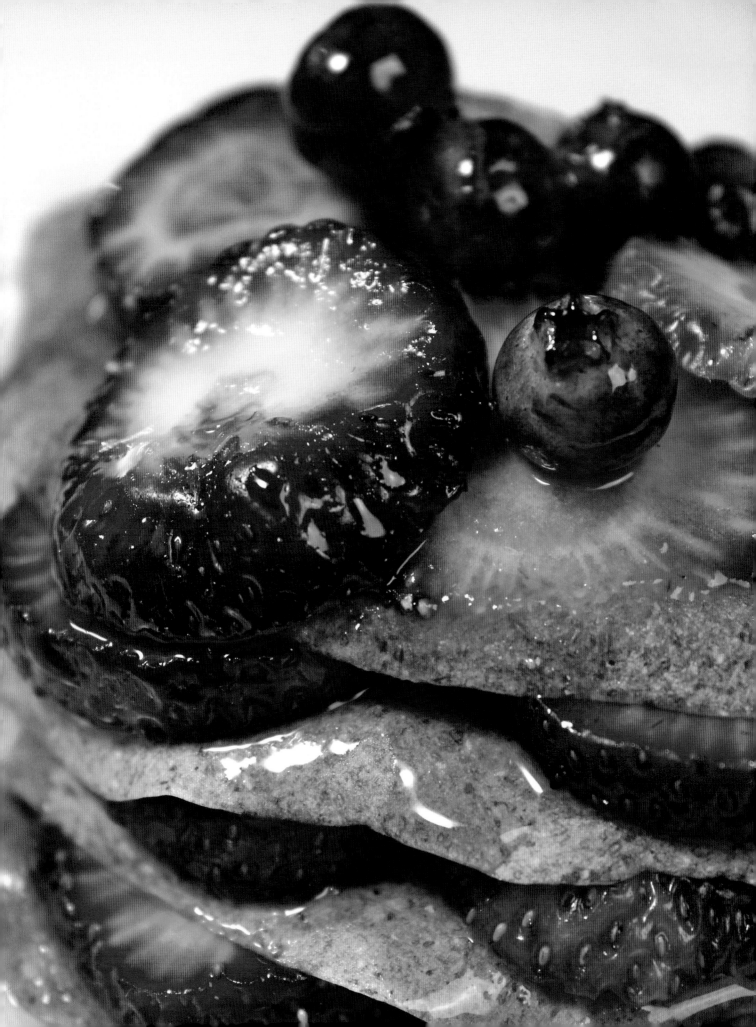

Breakfast (Frühstück)

German Green Drink with Apples, Almond Milk, and Cinnamon

2 cups almond milk (see p. 65)

2 apples, cored and chopped

⅛ teaspoon cinnamon

Pinch of nutmeg

Pinch of anise

Sweetener of choice

1 handful of dark leafy greens of choice

4 ice cubes

DIRECTIONS

Blend the ingredients in a high-speed blender.

Porridge with Fruit

1 cup oat groats, soaked overnight

1 teaspoon vanilla

1½ cups almond milk

2 tablespoons chia seeds

Pinch of salt

Maple syrup or sweetener of choice to taste

DIRECTIONS

In a pot on the stove, warm almond milk to body temperature. Turn off the flame, and add chia seeds stirring with wire whisk. Let seeds sit for 5 minutes, and whisk again. Add the remaining ingredients, and whisk in. Warm to body temperature again if needed, and continue whisking so the chia seeds do not clump up.

Topping

Choose peaches, apricots, apples, or any fruit in season you like. Chop or slice, and place on top of the porridge. Sprinkle cinnamon on top.

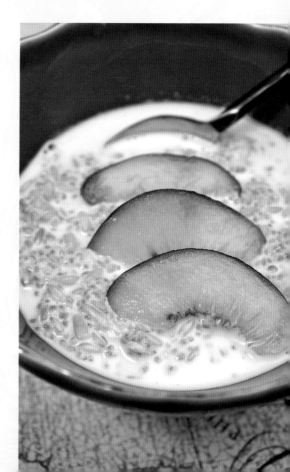

German Pancakes

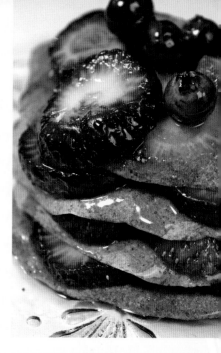

1 large ripe banana

1 cup cashews, soaked

1 cup pecans, soaked

1 tablespoon oat flour (see p. 45)

2 tablespoons almond milk

¼ cup maple syrup

1 small pinch cinnamon

1 pinch salt

¾ tablespoon vanilla

Extra maple syrup, for drizzling

DIRECTIONS

Place all ingredients in a high-speed blender. Scrape the sides down as necessary. Pour the mixture into a bowl, and stir with a spatula. Add more almond milk if necessary, one tablespoon at a time, to make a thick smooth batter, and stir well. Drop ¼ cup at a time on a nonstick dehydrator sheet to make a pancake shape. Tap the tray down on the kitchen counter to spread the pancake. The batter should make 6 pancakes. Dehydrate at 110° F for 2½ hours. Turn the nonstick sheet over onto a mesh sheet, and using a thin large knife, slowly lift the nonstick sheet while using a knife to loosen the pancake onto the mesh sheet. Dehydrate for another 1½ hours. Press down on the pancake with a finger to test readiness. It should be soft, but not sticky.

TO SERVE

Divide the pancakes on a plate, add fresh berries, and drizzle warm maple syrup on top.

Cardamom, Sunflower, and Caraway Seed Bread

A piece of good German bread spread with cheese makes a delicious breakfast (see p. 101 for cheese). A little drop of maple syrup or jam on top is also quite yummy.

1 cup wet almond pulp

1 cup sprouted buckwheat
  (see p. 44), ground to flour

½ cup flaxseed, finely ground

½ cup sunflower seeds, finely ground

½ cup psyllium, ground

2 cups young Thai coconut

5 Medjool dates, soaked to soften

6 cardamom pods, finely ground

½ teaspoon caraway seeds

1 clove garlic, crushed

1 cup water, or as needed

DIRECTIONS

Sprout the buckwheat. This will take 2–3 days until a little tail is noticed. Grind each of the following separately to powder: buckwheat, flaxseed, sunflower seeds, psyllium, ½ caraway seeds, and cardamom pods. When the ingredients are well-blended, place them in a food processor. Add the wet almond pulp to the processor.

Place the coconut meat, dates, garlic, and ½ cup water in a high-powered blender and blend well, adding more water a little at a time if

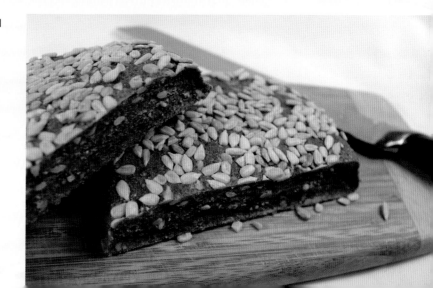

necessary to make a smooth mixture. Blend, stopping when needed to scrape down the sides. Pour the mixture into the food processor with other the ingredients, and pulse chop until incorporated. Place the dough into a bowl, and knead together with your hands to achieve a pliable texture. If the dough is dry, slowly add more water a tablespoon at a time. Divide the dough evenly into 2 pieces. Shape each piece into 2 firm loaves, about 2–3 inches high, and place them on a mesh dehydrator screen. Dehydrate at 115° F for 12–15 hours.

TIP { Sprinkle ¼ cup sunflower seeds on each loaf before dehydrating, and press them on top with your hands. This bread is so delicious served with good olive oil, crushed garlic, and a little salt. Mix the oil, garlic, and salt together, and dip the bread in.

Lunch (Mittagessen)

I love simple salads. They can be whipped up in minutes and are always satisfying. You can always add more ingredients, but something about a salad with a couple of good-quality greens or fruits allows each flavor to stand out. We found two buffets that happen to be in department stores with the most amazing salad fixings, including sprouts and seeds, and one restaurant even had a green drink. The top floor of KaDeWe, and the Galeria Kaufhof in an area called Alexanderplatz are not to be missed.

Arugula and Pear Salad

3–4 generous handfuls arugula, washed and spun dry

2 ripe pears, cored and thinly sliced (ripe pears are important to this salad)

¼ cup pecans, chopped

Dressing

1 teaspoon Dijon mustard	2–3 tablespoons extra-virgin olive oil
1 tablespoon apple cider vinegar	Himalayan salt to taste
1–2 teaspoons maple syrup	Freshly milled pepper to taste

DIRECTIONS
Whisk dressing together with a wire whisk.

TO SERVE
Place the washed and dried greens in a large salad bowl, and toss with half the dressing. Place on chilled plates. Toss sliced pears with the remaining dressing, and stack artfully on top of the greens. Chop the pecans, and sprinkle on top. You might also want to sprinkle some hemp seeds on top.

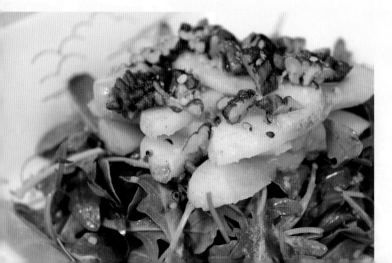

Beet and Carrot Salad

2 large beets, peeled, ends cut off   1 carrot, peeled, ends cut off

DIRECTIONS

Using a food processor, grate the beets and carrot separately, and place them in separate bowls.

Dressing

1 clove garlic, crushed

2 tablespoons tahini

3 tablespoons lemon juice

1 teaspoon apple cider vinegar

1 tablespoon extra-virgin olive oil

1 tablespoon maple syrup or sweetener of choice

Himalayan salt to taste

3–4 tablespoons water

DIRECTIONS

In a small bowl, add all ingredients except the water, and whisk together. Add water as necessary to make a smooth pourable dressing. Taste for seasonings, and adjust if necessary.

TO SERVE

Divide the dressing between the beets and carrot, and toss well. Mound each one separately on a plate, and garnish with sprouts.

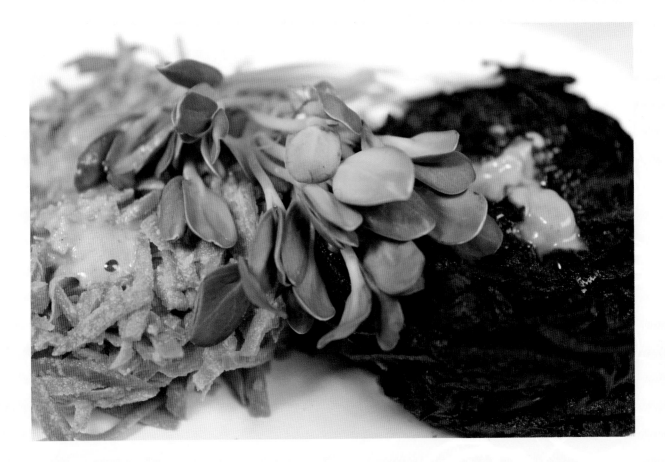

Dinner (Abendessen)

What would a German recipe section be without sausage? There are sausage stands all over Germany, serving a wide variety of wursts, all made with some kind of meat. I just couldn't resist trying my hand at this popular dish and make a raw vegan-style sausage. When they came out of the dehydrator, I was thrilled with the outcome. A little grainy mustard, and a new raw dish was born.

Sausage/Wurst

2½ cups sprouted wild rice (see p. 44)

1 cup walnuts

1 cup sunflower seeds, finely ground

1 cup carrot pulp made by juicing carrots

¼ cup sweet onion or shallot, which is milder

¼ cup parsley leaves, finely chopped

1 teaspoon caraway, ground

1 teaspoon summer savory

1½ teaspoons Dijon or homemade mustard (see p. 54)

½ teaspoon capers, crushed in garlic press

1 teaspoon tamari

1 tablespoon olive oil

Himalayan salt to taste

Freshly milled pepper to taste

¼ cup water, or more if needed

DIRECTIONS

Grind the sunflower seeds until very fine, and place in a mixing bowl. Place the sprouted rice and walnuts in a food processor, and grind well. Place the mixture in a bowl, and add the remaining ingredients. Mix well with a spatula. Add water as necessary so the mixture will stick together. Taste for seasonings, and adjust to your taste. If you have a juicer that has a blank plate, run everything through after mixing a couple of times.

TO SHAPE SAUSAGES

Measure ¼ cup of the mixture to make each sausage, place on a mesh screen, and roll back and forth on the screen to make the sausage shape. You should get 12 sausages from this mixture. Dehydrate at 115° F for 2½ –3½ hours. The sausages will have a crust on the outside and will be softer inside. Turn once during dehydration.

Mustard Sauce

¼ cup homemade or store-bought mustard (see p. 54)

Serve with Sauerkraut

½ head green cabbage

½ head purple cabbage

2 tablespoons Himalayan salt

1 teaspoon caraway seeds

1 teaspoon mustard seeds

DIRECTIONS

Pull 4 top leaves off your choice of cabbage which will be used for covering the shredded cabbage. Slice the cabbages as thinly as possible. This can be done by hand, with an attachment of a food processor, or with a mandolin slicer. Place the cabbage into a glass bowl, and sprinkle with salt. Massage

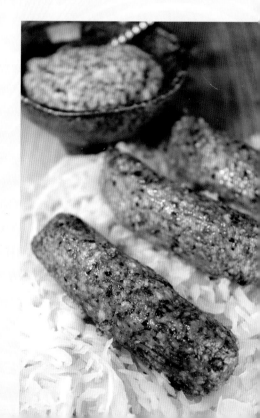

the cabbage to draw water out. Spend at least 5 minutes massaging. Put 1 cup water in, and place the reserved cabbage leaves on top to cover the shredded cabbage. Place a heavy weight on top to help press out the natural water from the cabbage. Cover with a cloth, and let sit. Check in 5 hours, and press down again. The cabbage should be under the waterline. Add more salt if you add more water. Check every day for 2 weeks, making sure the cabbage is under the waterline, and continue pushing down. When it tastes good to you, place it in clean glass jars and refrigerate.

Stuffed Cabbage with Tomato Sauce

(makes 16 stuffed cabbages)

16 cabbage leaves

2 cups jicama-cauliflower rice

1 cup parsley, finely chopped

2 tablespoons lemon juice

¼ cup small onion, finely chopped

½ cup zucchini, finely shredded

1 tablespoon dill

1 tablespoon caraway

1 tablespoon thyme

1 tablespoon marjoram

¼ teaspoon fennel seeds, finely crushed

1 tablespoon fresh mint, finely chopped

¼ cup currants

1 tablespoon extra-virgin olive oil

1 clove garlic, crushed

Himalayan salt to taste

Freshly milled pepper to taste

½ cup pine nuts

2 tablespoons water

DIRECTIONS

Remove the core of the cabbage, and carefully remove the leaves. This recipe makes 16 stuffed cabbages. With a paring knife, peel down the hard core on each leaf as flat as possible. Massage the leaves with olive-oiled hands, and lay them on a mesh dehydrator sheet. Dehydrate at 110° F for approximately 1 hour to wilt the leaves. Pulse chop the cauliflower in a food processor until it reaches fine rice texture. Remove, and chop jicama in the food processor until it reaches fine rice texture. Place both on a dehydrator sheet, and dehydrate for 1½ hours. When finished, transfer to a mixing bowl, and add the remaining ingredients, mixing until well incorporated. Taste for seasonings, and adjust to your liking.

HOW TO STUFF LEAVES

With the bottom end of a leaf on your left side, lay the leaf flat on a chopping board or plate. Place ¼ cup filling on the side of the leaf closest to you, and roll over once to cover the filling. Fold in the sides over the roll, and continue rolling firmly to make a closed package. Roll all cabbage leaves, and place in a glass baking dish. Cover with sauce. Cover the dish with foil, and dehydrate at 110° F for 3 hours.

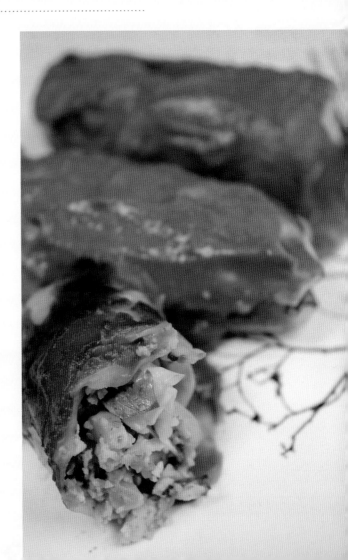

Sauce

2 ripe tomatoes, coarsely chopped

⅓ cup sun-dried tomato, soaked until soft

1 tablespoon olive oil

1 teaspoon thyme

1 teaspoon marjoram

Dash of maple syrup

Salt and pepper to taste

DIRECTIONS

Blend all ingredients until smooth, adding water a little at a time if necessary. Add on top of the cabbage leaves halfway through dehydration, or warm separately to pour on top of the finished rolls. Serve warm or at room temperature.

Sweet Potato Noodles with Cheesy Cheese Sauce

Germans love their potatoes, but white potatoes are one dish that is just not good raw. However, sweet potatoes lend themselves very well to raw dishes.

NOODLES

2 sweet potatoes, spiral cut (use potato peeler if you do not own spiralizer)

CHEEZY CHEESE SAUCE

2 cups raw cashews, soaked for 4 hours

4 tablespoons lemon juice

1½ cups water

⅛ cup olive oil

2–3 tablespoons fresh rosemary, minced

3 teaspoons gluten-free tamari

3 tablespoons nutritional yeast

1 teaspoon Himalayan salt or to taste

Ground black pepper to taste

DIRECTIONS

Place all ingredients into a high-speed blender, and blend into thick cream, adding water as needed. Taste for seasonings, and add more to your liking. Garlic can also be added along with ribbon-cut basil to garnish.

TIP { This dish can be warmed in a pan on the stove to body temperature. The noodles will relax and become softer.

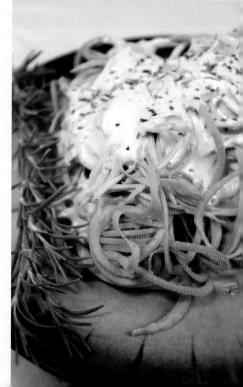

Dessert (Nachspeise)
German Chocolate Cake

(This recipe makes one six-inch double layer cake, using removable bottom form, and one five-inch one, using removable bottom form.)

Raw cakes are dense, especially this one. A very thin slice will be sufficient to satisfy almost anyone. You can make 8–10 slices from the six-inch cake.

This is a rich dark chocolate cake. If you want a full-size two-layer cake, double the recipe and frosting, and frost between the layers as well as the outside of the cake. The cake will last around 3 days refrigerated or may be frozen for a longer period of time.

1 cup almonds, ground into flour (see p. 45)

1 cup hazelnuts, ground into flour

1 cup pecans, ground into flour

1 teaspoon vanilla

¼ cup cacao powder

2 tablespoons coconut oil

¼ cup almond milk

15 Medjool dates, soaked until soft and made into paste in food processor

Pinch of Himalayan salt

DIRECTIONS

Pull out your electric hand mixer. Place all ingredients in a large mixing bowl, and on low speed whip lightly to incorporate all ingredients. Continue mixing, gradually turning up the speed. The purpose is to break up all the lumps and make fluffier dough.

Rub a light coat of coconut oil on the pans. Place half of the cake mixture into the pans, pushing only lightly to hold together; do not press hard. Save half for the second layer. Place in a freezer while you make the filling/frosting.

FILLING/FROSTING LAYER

2 cups walnuts

1 cup large coconut flakes

½ cup maple syrup or sweetener of choice

1 tablespoon coconut oil

1 teaspoon vanilla extract

¼ cup small coconut flakes, plus 2 tablespoons reserved for topping

DIRECTIONS

Mix all ingredients together in a food processor except the small coconut flakes until completely smooth, scraping down the sides as needed. Scrape into a bowl, and mix in the small flakes. Spread a thin layer of frosting on the first cake layer. Use hands if necessary, keeping them slightly wet to spread the mixture. Place the second layer of cake mixture on top of the frosting. Finish off with a balance of frosting, and sprinkle with large and fine coconut pieces.

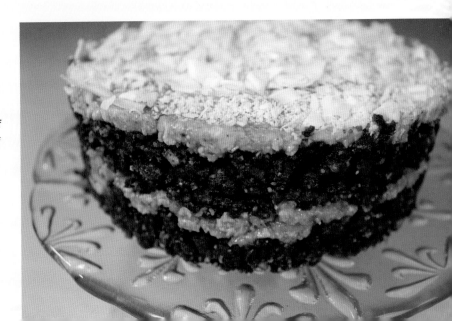

Apple Strudel

DOUGH

1 cup macadamia nuts or almonds, made into flour

½ cup wet almond pulp

1 cup coconut or almond flour

1 cups young Thai coconut meat

½ cup almond milk, or more if necessary

¼ cup flaxseed, finely ground

6 Medjool dates, soaked to soften

3–4 tablespoons maple syrup or sweetener of choice

½ teaspoon cinnamon

Dash of nutmeg

Pinch of Himalayan salt

DIRECTIONS

Grind the nuts to powder. Place in a bowl. Add the coconut flour and wet almond pulp, and mix. Place the coconut meat and dates in a blender with the almond milk, and blend until smooth. Pour into a bowl with dry ingredients, and mix until all ingredients are well incorporated. The mixture should be dough-like. Press out on a nonstick dehydrator sheet, and use a rolling pin to make a flat piece of dough approximately 10" × 11". Dehydrate for 1 hour at 115° F while making the filling.

Filling

1 cup dried apples*, soaked in 2 cups apple juice to reconstitute

2 cups fresh apples, coarsely chopped and tossed with 1 tablespoon lemon juice

6 Medjool dates, soaked until soft

2 ounces Irish moss gel (see p. 46)

½ teaspoon cinnamon

⅛ teaspoon nutmeg

3 tablespoons maple syrup or sweetener of choice

1 teaspoon vanilla

Pinch of Himalayan sea salt

*You could dry apples in a dehydrator, or you could purchase organic, naturally dried apples from the farmers market, health food store, or online.

DIRECTIONS

When dried apples are hydrated, strain the juice to make Irish moss gel. Place the chopped moss in a blender with 1½ cups apple juice. Make more juice if necessary. Blend adding water, if needed, to make a thick gel. Be sure the mixture is completely smooth and thick and any small pieces of Irish moss are dissolved.

In a food processor, place the chopped fresh apples, Irish moss gel, Medjool dates, cinnamon, nutmeg, sweetener, vanilla, salt, and blend until smooth.

In a mixing bowl, combine the apple mixture from the food processor together with the hydrated apples, and blend with a spatula until well incorporated. Raisins that have been soaked and softened may be added at this time if desired. Taste for sweetness, and add more sweetener if necessary.

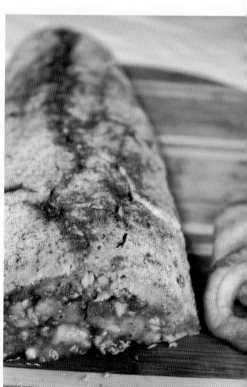

TO ASSEMBLE

Here is where the artistry in you comes into play. Treat the dough like a piece of clay. If you've never worked with wet clay, it's very forgiving and pliable. After one hour of dehydration, the dough will be ready to work with. Place the filling down the middle of the dough, lengthwise. Using a pastry spatula (if you have one) or a large chopping knife, gently lift one side over the apples and then the other side over the top. Use your hands to shape the strudel. Wet your hands and heal any cracks in the dough; press and work the dough until it is sealed and compact. Don't worry about small imperfections, as this is a rustic strudel. Place back in the dehydrator at 110° F, brush with melted coconut oil, and dehydrate for 8–9 more hours. Slice with a bread knife for best results. Serve with a drizzle of maple syrup.

Spice Cookie

2 cups cashew flour (see p. 45)

1 cup oat flour

1 cup wet almond pulp (see p. 65)

1 ripe banana

⅓ cup maple sugar

2 Medjool dates or 1 tablespoon coconut sugar

½ cup unsweetened coconut flakes, medium size

½ generous cup currants or raisins, soaked until soft

¼ teaspoon cinnamon

⅛ teaspoon nutmeg

⅛ teaspoon ground clove

¼ teaspoon ground cardamom

½ cup walnut pieces for topping

DIRECTIONS

In a food processor, place the flours, almond pulp, banana, and sweeteners. Pulse chop until everything is blended in. Place the mixture in a mixing bowl, and add the coconut, raisins, and spices. Use a cookie scooper, and place a scoop on a nonstick sheet of a dehydrator tray. This shape will be rounded. You can also press down for a standard-looking cookie. Press the walnut pieces on top of the cookie. Dehydrate at 115° F for 10–12 hours or more, depending on how dry you like them. Remove halfway through drying, and place on mesh dehydrator sheets. I prefer a light crust on the outside and a small part of the center softer. The cookie tastes great warm right from the dehydrator with a cold glass of almond milk.

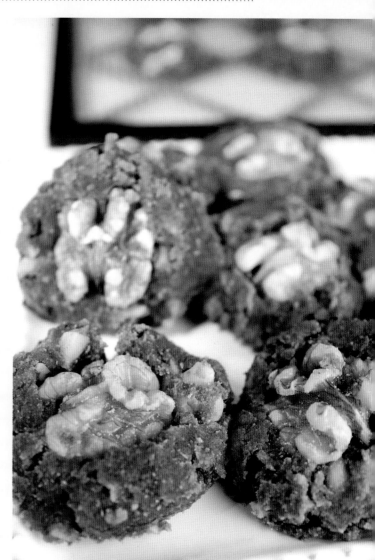

Drinks (Getränke)

Germans love their beer, but they also love nonalcoholic beverages, including vitamin-laden fruit drinks. There wasn't a country we traveled to that did not love coffee, but we were amazed to see how much Germany loved its aromatic fruit juices, including apple juice served with sparkling water; orange juice; apple-pear, apple-mango, or apple-grape juice; and multivitamin juice with tropical blends. Germans have a list of "wellness drinks" that contain antioxidants; vitamins A, C, and E; and omega-3 fatty acids. It was a surprise to learn that soda is not as popular as it is in America.

Apple Juice Tea

2 cups apple juice, freshly squeezed

1½ cups green tea, freshly brewed

Juice from ½ lemon

Juice from ½ orange

Dash of cinnamon

Dash of cloves

Maple syrup, or sweetener of choice, to taste

DIRECTIONS

Mix all ingredients together, then warm to body temperature or place in a glass with ice.

Fruit Spritzer

Any fresh fruit juice can turn into a spritzer. All you need is fresh juice, carbonated water, sweetener, and ice.

Cranberry Spritzer

1 cup fresh or frozen cranberries

Sweetener of choice to taste

1 cup water

DIRECTIONS

Blend the ingredients in a high-powered blender until completely smooth. Strain the mixture through a cheesecloth, nut filter bag, or sieve. Taste for sweetness, and add more sweetener if necessary. Place ice in a glass and pour juice over it, filing the glass about three quarters. Add sparkling water to top the glass. Stir, and garnish with lemon peel or a celery leaf.

SUGGESTIONS

Substitute cranberries with orange, grape, lemon, lime, and pineapple pieces.

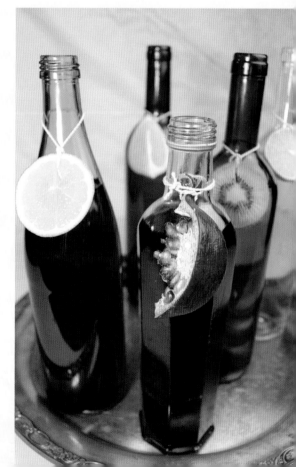

Medieval Spiced Drink

In the Middle Ages, water was often unclean, so the poor drank ale or cider whereas the rich drank wine. Beer, one of Germany's favorite drinks, is one of the oldest fermented beverages and was popular in medieval times. Fermented food is one of the best foods for our gut, and this recipe might help promote some good bacteria in your system.

12 organic apples

Sweetener of choice

Mulling herbs can be purchased ready, or make your own from the following:

1 cinnamon stick

2 pieces star anise

⅛ teaspoon nutmeg

⅛ teaspoon fresh ginger

⅛ teaspoon allspice, whole if possible

⅛ teaspoon cardamom pods

4 whole cloves

Rind of 1 orange and 1 lemon

Water as needed

DIRECTIONS

Core and seed the 6 apples, and put them through the homogenizing blade of a juicer or mash them in a food processor. Place the apples in a bowl, then press and squeeze them to release any juices. Add the mulling herbs. Juice the balance of the apples, and pour into a bowl; mix well. Transfer to a large jar or two, and add water to make a tea consistency. Lay a paper towel or cheesecloth over the opening of the jar, and secure with a rubber band. Leave the mixture on the kitchen counter for 2 days. Strain the mixture, and juice the balance of liquid in a high-speed blender. Taste, and add sweetener if necessary. Refrigerate, and serve chilled.

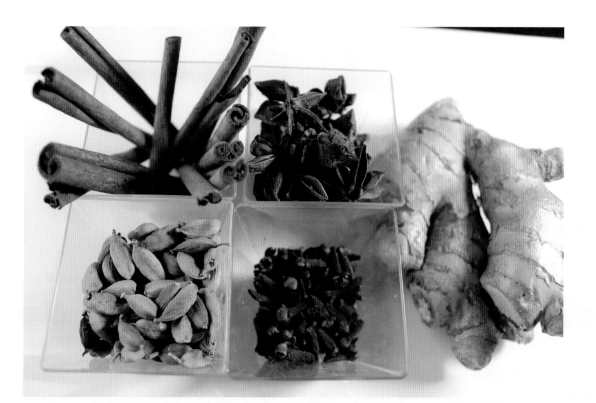

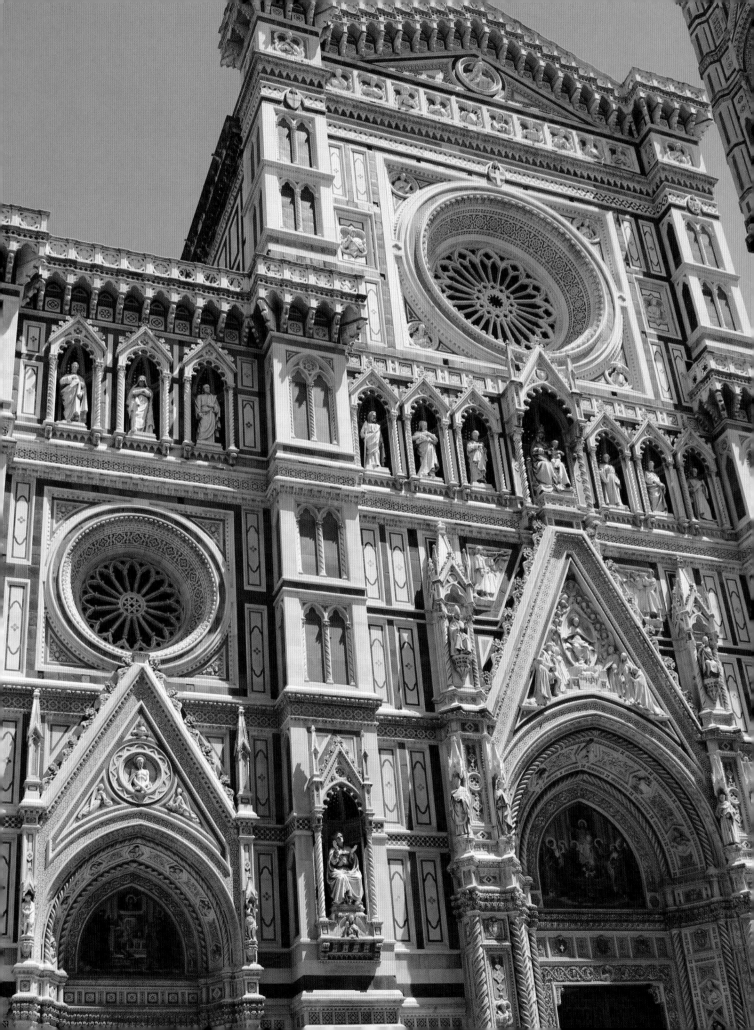

I've probably traveled to Italy more than any other country abroad. I fell in love with it the first time I visited in the early seventies, when I worked for the actress Valerie Harper. Years later, with some travel mileage under my belt, I traveled alone to Italy for my sixtieth birthday. On that trip I met some lifelong Italian friends. This was the first time I traveled abroad alone. I rented a lovely inexpensive small room online, flew into Rome, and took a train from the airport to Florence. It was quite an adventure not speaking the language and trying to figure out which train I should be on. I was a little tired from the long trip from California but very excited to be in Florence. I somehow found my hotel, took the ancient elevator to my room, put down my bag, and immediately opened the window, which faced a lovely courtyard full of flowers. I unpacked my bag and put my clothes away in the tiny dresser, and as tired as I was, I left my room to walk the city for hours. Florence is such a romantic city and even more so at night. Several younger men flirted with me, which of course made me feel lovely. It seems like the Italian men love all women, of any age.

For my actual birthday I took a train for the day to Venice. Little did I know that one day in Venice would not be nearly enough. When it was time to catch the last train back to Florence, I just couldn't leave. Since I kept my hotel in Florence and didn't bring any of my belongings, I needed to find a room and some necessities. Venice was packed, but I managed to find a beautiful little hotel that had one room left. It was a very tiny room with a twin-size bed. No wonder it was vacant—how many people travel to Venice alone? I went for some emergency shopping to pick up toiletries, underwear, and a new blouse. I celebrated my birthday dinner in a restaurant with no English-speaking service. At that time I didn't speak any Italian, but it didn't seem to matter; we seemed to understand each other well enough. I celebrated myself—sixty needs a good celebration, and a couple of glasses of red wine were in order. After dinner, I strolled the streets of Venice discovering little nooks and crannies of delights. I knew I would return to Venice again. The next day I walked for hours and reluctantly hopped on the last train back to Florence. It was the perfect birthday! It was a perfect trip. I tell you this story only to encourage you to be bold. Don't wait for others if there is no one around to travel with; go by yourself and be open to a new adventure.

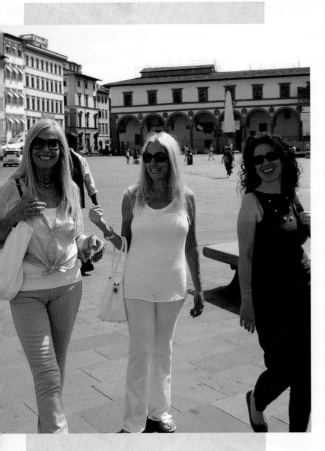

I've traveled to Italy many times over the years, and I've never tired of it. In fact, I just can't seem to get enough. On this trip, the book-writing tour with Mike and our friends, Michael and Eileen, with whom we met up in Florence, Italy was extra special. Working on this book while traveling gave us all such pleasure. We never lacked for delicious meals. The farmers markets have everything we needed. You can find ambrosia-tasting tomatoes of every shape and variety and each more delicious and juicy than the last. Add a little basil and great olive oil, and nothing could taste better. I chose this meal many times in restaurants and always felt satisfied. Greens are everywhere and not just at farmers markets; supermarkets are full of dark leafy greens.

When we travel to Rome, we usually visit our very dear friend Monica Mazzitelli, who is a great host and tour guide as she was born in Rome. She introduced us to a salad restaurant called Ensalada Ricca, which I though worth mentioning in case you travel to Rome. We've enjoyed their salads many times on previous trips. Since we did not have time for Rome on this trip, Monica met up with us in Florence. She is amazingly fun to be with, and I always learn something new from her about Italy. As much as I like to try out my Italian, it's always so much easier when Monica does the talking to locals.

My love for Italian food is obvious, and many Italian recipes were included in *Live Raw*, but the delights of Italian food never end, and on this trip I discovered more delicacies, which you will find in this chapter. Italian food is made with simple fresh ingredients, allowing the taste to shine through. Italy is where I learned that the freshness of ingredients could make or break a meal.

As luck would have it, Donna Brown, author of *Food & Flowers* and *Happy Food*, contacted me and invited us all to her organic olive oil farm, called Campo di Torri, which is a magical villa with rolling vineyards and mountain views. It is located just a short train ride outside Florence. Just a drop of her farm's olive oil drizzled on a ripe tomato is pure ambrosia.

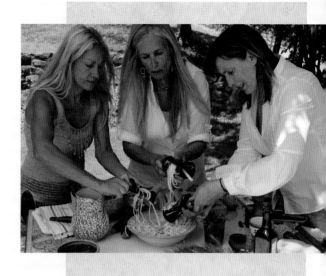

Donna and her husband, Eduardo Salvia, live in Milan most of the year and travel to their farm for relaxation and work. Donna and I planned a great day together. We thought we could fix a raw meal for her family and my traveling companions. I e-mailed her a grocery list, which was followed by many back and forth online discussions. We arrived by train from Florence, and Donna met us at the station and took us to her farm. This experience was one of the loveliest parts of our trip. Out by the pool, on a beautiful large table, we prepared zucchini pasta, a cool summer soup, and banana ice cream with fresh berries. Our all-raw lunch was quite delicious, and even the Italians were amazed at how good the pasta tasted. Eduardo said it was one of the best pasta dishes he ever had. That is a huge compliment coming from someone from Naples, who didn't expect much from uncooked zucchini pasta. Donna and I had lots to share about what it takes to write a cookbook, as she was just finishing her second book, *Happy Food*. We had fun exchanging food and plating tips, at which she is an expert. Eduardo, who is as passionate as anyone could be about his olive trees and spices, showed us how olive oil is made. We came away with unforgettable memories of a wonderful day, with gifts of olive oil and herbs and new friends that I can't wait to spend time with again.

Mike, Michael, Eileen, and I traveled to small hilltop towns, visited friends, soaked up farmers markets, picked herbs, and took photographs everywhere we went. We also spent a few days with my good friend Robin Leach and his son Steve. Robin spends a few weeks in Italy every summer. Eileen and I fixed a raw food dinner one evening, and we all enjoyed a delicious meal alfresco with warm winds and cold champagne. Some of the food we prepared came straight out of the gardens the owners maintain for guests of the villa Robin rents. There's nothing like life under the Tuscan sun and, as Robin always says, "Il dolce far niente," the sweetness of doing nothing.

grow your own italian herb garden

No yard? No problem. Start your Italian garden in pots. Container gardens are very successful and easy to care for. A good watering system, sunshine, and love, and you have yourself a garden. In Italy you will find herbs growing in pots on balconies, on porches, and at front doors. In any corner where a pot will fit and get a little sun, you will find something growing. Buy heirloom seeds if possible, or skip that step and buy organic starter plants.

Good organic-growing soil designed for container gardening is very important. Containers dry out quickly, so check daily to learn the watering needs of the plants. You can start your seeds in a small container indoors, then transplant into larger containers outside.

TYPICAL ITALIAN HERB GARDEN

Basil, rosemary, oregano, thyme, garlic, sage, and if you have room, tomatoes are essential to Italian dishes and fun to grow.

Depending on the room you have available, the potted plants of these six herbs will not take up much room or much of your time, but they will give you a gigantic amount of pleasure and add spice to your life.

ITALIAN HERBS AND SPICES

Italian herbs pair well with tomato-based sauces, breads, soups, salad dressings, stews, and pizzas. For a mixed blend, combine equal amounts of basil, thyme, marjoram, oregano, and Italian flat parsley, and a smaller amount of rosemary and sage. Dry the herbs to mix them together and keep on hand, or use fresh herbs when possible.

Buon Appetito (Enjoy Your Meal)

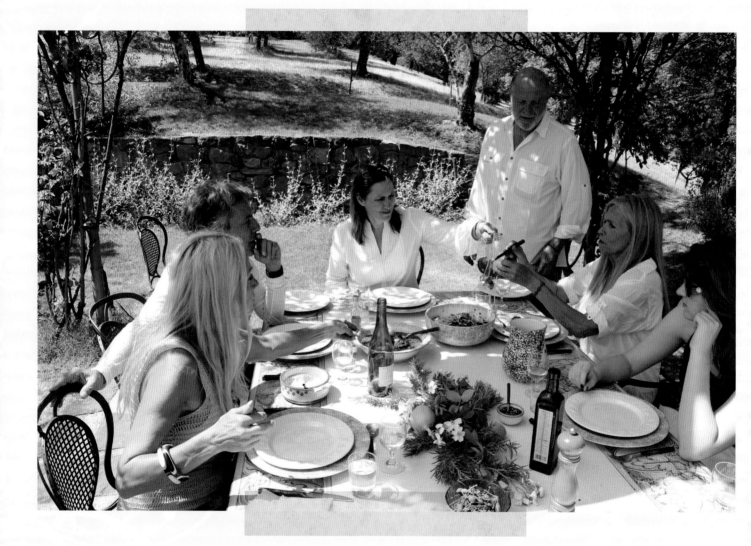

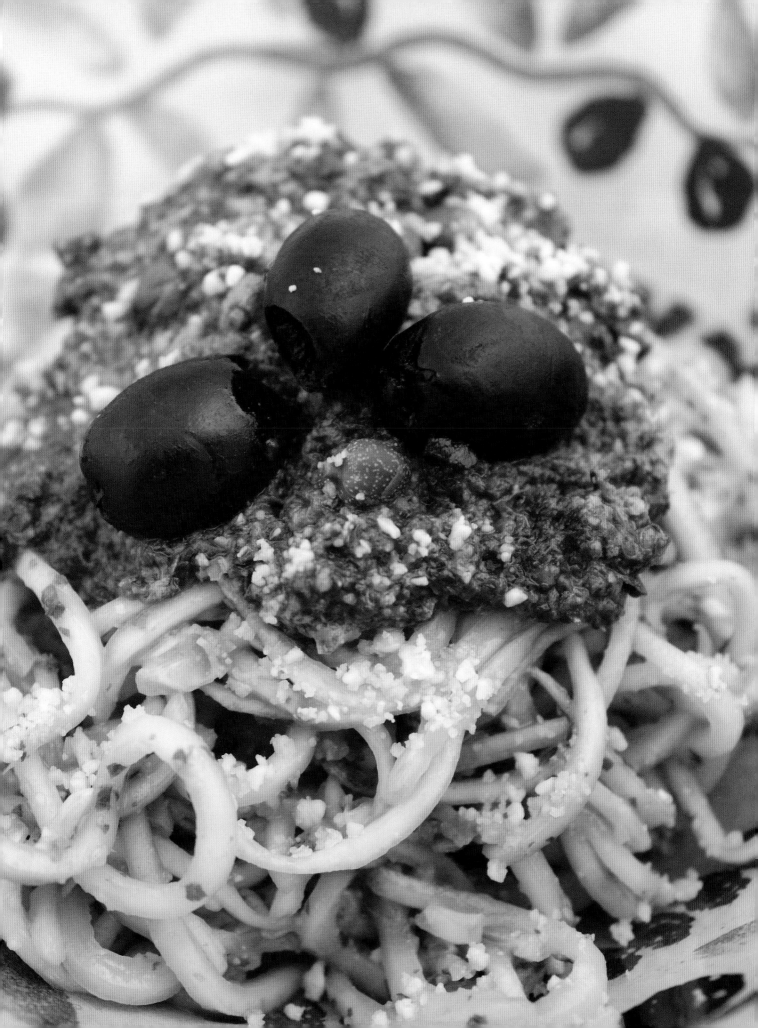

Breakfast (Colazione)

Most Italians have coffee for breakfast accompanied by bread or some sort of sweet roll. I don't see Italians eating eggs and the kinds of breakfast we see in America, except in tourist hotels. It's true Italians like sweets for breakfast.

Italian Green Smoothie

(2 servings)

   In keeping with the spirit of sweets and simplicity for breakfast, this green drink will fit right into the Italian style.

2 cups spinach	3 Medjool dates
1–2 apples	Water to desired consistency
1 cup berries of any kind	Lots of ice
3 fresh or dried figs	

DIRECTIONS

Place all ingredients in a high-speed blender, adding water as needed. Blend until smooth consistency is reached. On a warm day, pour over ice and add a squeeze of lemon.

Cappuccino with Cashew Milk

So rich and creamy, you won't even know it's not the real thing.

1 cup cashews, soaked for 2–4 hours	2 teaspoons cacao powder
3½ cups water	Dash of cinnamon
3 Medjool dates, soaked, or 2 tablespoons coconut sugar	½ vanilla pod, chopped
2 teaspoons maca	2 tablespoons coconut oil

I usually recommend that people not drink coffee, but if you would like to, you can add coffee extract to this cappuccino (see p. 66), or you can make a very low acidic version by putting 3–4 tablespoons ground organic coffee in ½ cup warmed water overnight. When ready to use, strain through a filter, and use a tablespoon or two in the cappuccino.

DIRECTIONS

Drain the cashews, and place them in a blender with pure fresh water. After blending until smooth, remove 1 tablespoon and place in a small bowl. This will be used for the topping. Add the remaining ingredients to the blender, and blend very well. Adjust the consistency with water; some like it thick, and some like it thin. Add more sweetener to your liking. Cappuccino may be warmed on the stove to body temperature or iced on a warm day.

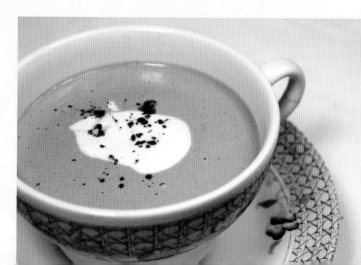

Pour it into your favorite cup, and top with reserved cashew cream. Sprinkle a bit of cacao powder on top. Mamma mia, so delizioso!

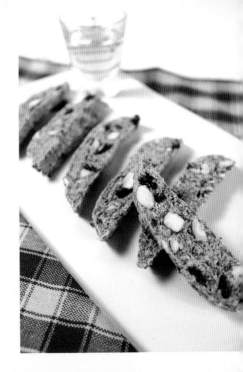

Almond Biscotti with Anise Seeds

2 cups almond flour (see p. 45)

1 cup oat groat flour (see p. 45)

½ cup young Thai coconut meat

¼ cup flax meal

1 teaspoon almond extract

½ teaspoon hazelnut extract

⅓ cup almonds, chopped

½ cup maple syrup or sweetener of choice

Orange juice as needed for moisture

1 teaspoon anise seeds

¼ cup currants

DIRECTIONS

Place the almond flour, oat groat flour, and flax meal in a food processor, pulse chop until blended, and transfer the mixture to a mixing bowl. In a high-speed blender, place the coconut meat, sweetener, ¼ cup orange juice, and extract. Blend until very smooth. Pour into the bowl with the dry mixture. Add nuts and anise seed, blending with a spatula, adding more orange juice as needed to make semifirm dough. On a nonstick dehydrator sheet, shape the dough into a long loaf about 2 inches high. Dehydrate at 110° F for 4–5 hours. Cut into biscotti-size pieces with a sharp knife or serrated bread knife, lay flat on a mesh screen, and dehydrate another for 8–10 hours until completely dry.

Chocolate Zucchini Bread

2 cups zucchini, unpeeled and grated

1 cup wet almond pulp

2 tablespoons chia seeds, finely ground

3 tablespoons flaxseeds, finely ground to meal

¼ cup psyllium meal

2 tablespoons extra-virgin olive oil

½ cup maple syrup, or sweeter of choice

1 tablespoon vanilla

½ cup Medjool dates, chopped

⅛ teaspoon cinnamon

5 tablespoons cacao powder

Pinch of Himalayan salt

Water as necessary

DIRECTIONS

Grate or grind the zucchini in a food processor. Transfer into a mixing bowl. Place the almond pulp, flaxseeds, chia seeds, and psyllium in the food processor, and pulse chop until well incorporated. Place in the mixing bowl containing the zucchini. Add olive oil, sweetener, dates, cinnamon, cacao powder, and salt to the bowl. Blend well to make dough. Taste for sweetness, and add more sweetener if necessary. Divide the dough into 2 balls, and shape each into a loaf. Place the loaves on a mesh screen, and dehydrate at 110—115° F for 20–24 hours. Serve with jam (see pp. 53-54).

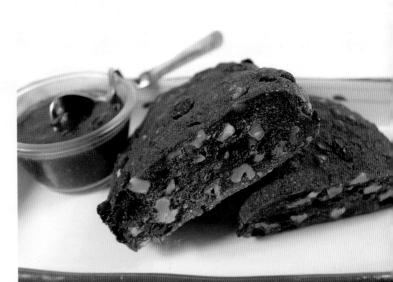

Lunch (Pranzo)
Zucchini Pasta with Creamy Pesto Puttanesca

(2–3 servings)

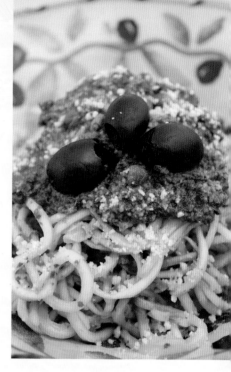

This versatile pasta dish can be eaten for lunch or dinner. Many sauces work well, but this particular one is yummy.

PASTA

3 large, straight zucchinis

DIRECTIONS

Peel the skin off the zucchinis or leave it on—your choice. Run through the spiralizer on a thin pasta blade, or use a potato peeler for fettuccini noodles. Break or cut strings if they are too long. Place the zucchini pasta in a large bowl, and massage with a little oil and lemon. Let it rest for about 10–15 minutes to soften, then massage again. Pour off any liquid.

Pesto

2 cups packed basil leaves	Freshly milled pepper to taste
½ cup walnuts or pine nuts	⅛ teaspoon dried chili flakes, or to taste
3 tablespoons extra-virgin olive oil	2 tablespoons capers, crushed in garlic press
1 large clove garlic	
½ cup parsley leaves	1 tablespoon capers, whole
Himalayan salt	½ cup olives, raw if possible

DIRECTIONS

Place the basil, nuts, garlic, salt, and pepper in a food processor, and pulse chop. Drizzle in olive oil while the blender is running. Stop, scrap down the sides, and taste. Adjust with salt and pepper to your liking. Add more olive oil to make the pesto creamy. Smooth, thick, and pourable is what you are looking for. Add chili flakes if desired, and stir. Remove the pesto from the processor, and add a squeeze of lemon. Mix, and taste again for spices.

Parmesan Cheese

1 cup cashews	Himalayan salt to taste
1 clove garlic	

DIRECTIONS

Place all ingredients in a food processor, and pulse chop until the pieces are small and resemble Parmesan cheese. Do not overprocess or the cashews will turn to butter. Taste, and add more salt if desired. Store in an airtight container in a refrigerator.

TO ASSEMBLE

Toss the zucchini pasta in the pesto sauce, capers, and olives. Taste, and adjust with salt and pepper to your liking. Sprinkle cashew Parmesan cheese on top, and serve warm or at room temperature.

Antipasto Pinzimonio

Not only does this dish make a spectacular presentation, but is also only takes a short time to prepare. Antipasto Pinzimonio can be served at lunch or as a starter for dinner. I was quite surprised many years ago when I found a dish called pinzimonio on many menus in Italy. Pinzimonio, which means "fresh raw vegetables," is sometimes presented in a large serving bowl with a sharp knife or two. The vegetables are left whole or cut into large chunks. Personally, I love the look of the whole vegetables as it makes me feel as if I were living in Roman times (or at least that's what is depicted in films). Each person is given a small bowl, in which he or she can mix his or her own delicious rich olive oil, balsamic vinegar, salt, and pepper to taste. On many platters you'll find a small artichoke, which you eat in the same manner you would a cooked artichoke. The artichokes were good raw in Italy, but I've never found an artichoke that I like raw in the United States, except if the heart is sliced very thin for a salad. I admit, I allow myself a steamed artichoke on occasion.

PINZIMONIO

(2–3 Servings)

½ head of cauliflower	½ bunch of celery
1 red and 1 orange bell pepper	Several radishes
1 cucumber	½ fennel bulb
3 carrots	

DIPPING SAUCE

½ cup cold-pressed virgin olive oil	Freshly milled pepper to taste
1 teaspoon Himalayan salt	Aged balsamic vinegar (optional)

DIRECTIONS

Blend the olive oil, salt, and pepper in a small bowl. Arrange the vegetables on a large platter. Place the dipping sauce in small individual bowls for each guest, or you can put olive oil, salt, and pepper on the table and have the guests mix their own to their liking. It's hard not to double-dip this simple Italian summer favorite. Add some raw olives, a glass of wine if you indulge, a CD of Andrea Bocelli, and a table outdoors, and you are instantly transported to the countryside of Italy.

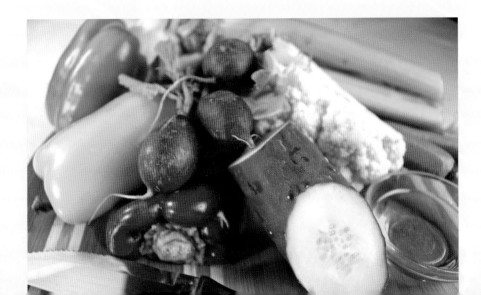

Minestrone Soup

BROTH

2½ cups tomato, seeded and cut in chunks

¾ cup sun-dried tomatoes, soaked until soft

1 carrot, peeled and cut in chunks

2 stalks celery, cut in chunks

2 cloves garlic

2 cups water (use tomato-soaking water)

½ teaspoon rosemary

2 tablespoons oregano or mixed Italian herbs

2 tablespoons olive oil

Himalayan salt to taste

Pepper to taste

DIRECTIONS

Blend the sun-dried tomatoes, water, herbs, salt, and pepper, but leave the mixture a little chunky. Place it in a food processor with the fresh tomatoes and balance of ingredients and blend, leaving the mixture a little chunky. Add water as needed to reach the desired consistency.

Vegetables

1 large zucchini, spiral-cut into pasta noodles, or use potato peeler to make strips

1 carrot, chopped

½ cup corn, cut off the cob

½ cup basil, chopped

1 tablespoon pesto (optional)

TO SERVE

Chop the noodles into 2–3-inch pieces. Toss the carrot in oil and dehydrate it for 1 hour, or use as is for the crunch. Warm the broth in a bowl placed over a pan of boiling water, heat it in a pan to body temperature, or use a dehydrator. Place chopped and spiral-cut vegetables in serving bowls. Pour the warm soup broth over the vegetables, and drizzle with some good olive. Sprinkle with cashew Parmesan cheese (see p. 140).

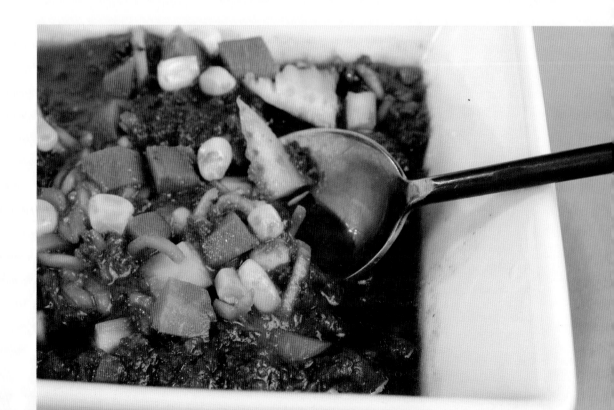

Dinner (Cena)

Italian Herb-Stuffed Sweet Red Pepper

2 sweet red bell peppers, cut lengthwise in half and seeded

1½ cups sprouted wild rice (see recipe below)

1 cup walnuts

Himalayan salt

Freshly ground pepper to taste

2 tablespoons Italian herbs

1 stalk celery, finely chopped

½ cup wet almond pulp

¼–½ sweet onion, finely chopped

2–3 tablespoons homemade ketchup (see p. 54), or purchase organic ketchup if necessary

DIRECTIONS

Pulse chop the rice and walnuts in a food processor to a medium grind, reserving ½ cup whole wild rice. Place the chopped rice mixture, whole rice, chopped onions, celery, and Italian herbs in a bowl, and combine well. Add salt, pepper, and wet almond pulp, and blend in. Add 2–3 tablespoons homemade catsup, and blend. Taste for salt and pepper, and adjust if necessary.

Stuff each pepper to fill its cavity. Put 1 inch of water and 1 tablespoon olive oil in a small glass baking dish just large enough to hold the peppers. Place the peppers in the dish, and top each pepper with ketchup. Cover with foil, and place in a dehydrator at 110° F for 3–4 hours. If you must use an oven, set on the lowest temperature with the door ajar, and warm for 10–15 minutes, taking care not to cook or overheat. Test by touching the skin of the peppers to see if it is warm and starting to wilt. The internal temperature of the peppers will not be affected if you keep an eye on them and do not overheat them.

Sprouted Wild Rice

Place 1 cup rinsed wild rice in a mason jar. Fill the jar with water, and cover with the lid. Place the jar in a dehydrator at 105°F, and in the morning you will have sprouted rice.

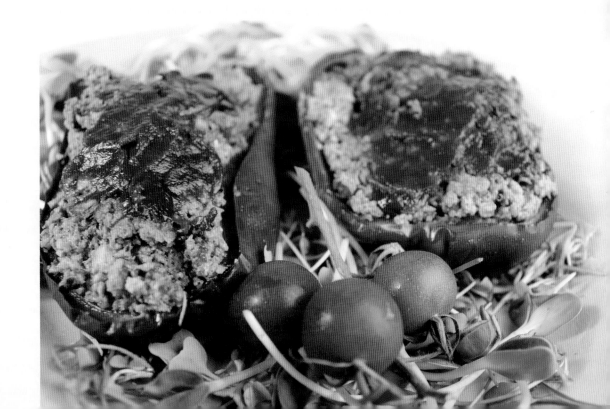

Mushrooms alla Parmigiana

In Italy it's easy to find lasagna or eggplant Parmesan, but those of us looking for healthier alternatives will be happy with the taste of this portobello mushroom Parmesan. The warm melting nut cheese paired with the marinated mushrooms and topped with a slice of lightly dehydrated tomato and pesto will certainly satisfy any cravings.

2 large portobello mushrooms

1 cup macadamia or cashew cheese (see p. 19)

½ cup cashew Parmesan (see p. 140)

1 large red pepper

3 sun-dried tomato halves, soaked until soft

½ zucchini, thinly sliced on mandolin slicer

Marinade

3 tablespoons tamari

2 tablespoons olive oil

3 tablespoons water

½ tablespoon Italian herbs

DIRECTIONS FOR MUSHROOMS, ZUCCHINI, AND TOMATOES

Wipe the mushroom clean with a damp paper towel. Remove the stems, and scrape the gills out with a melon baller or spoon. Slice off the curved ring around the mushroom caps with a sharp knife or serrated bread knife, leaving a solid piece of mushroom, and marinate for 20 minutes. Dehydrate at 110° F for 1–1½ hours. Marinate the zucchini and tomato, and place them on a dehydrator nonstick sheet to soften at 110° F for 1 hour.

DIRECTIONS FOR SAUCE

Seed and peel the red pepper with a potato peeler to remove as much skin as possible.
Cut in quarters, and dehydrate for 1–2 hours at 110–115° F to soften. When soft, place in a blender with the soaked tomato pieces and blend with a little water, salt, and pepper. Keep the mixture thick but smooth by adding only a tablespoon of water at a time.

TO ASSEMBLE

The mushrooms can be stacked for individual serving or layered in a glass baking dish. To start, spoon the sauce on the bottom of the dish. Arrange the mushrooms on top of the sauce. Layer cheese on top of mushroom, a large basil leaf, a dehydrated tomato, pesto, and zucchini slices. Sprinkle Parmesan cheese on top. If desired, the dish may be put back in a dehydrator to warm before serving. If using a baking dish, the mushrooms may be sliced and then layered in casserole style.

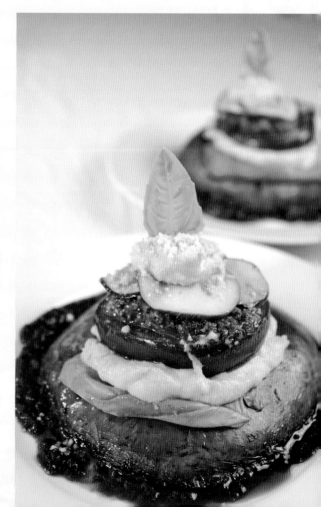

Wild Grass Risotto with Fresh Peas, Asparagus, and Pine Nut Cheese

(2–3 servings)

1 cup wild rice, to arrive at 2½ cups when sprouted (see p. 44)

1 cup freshly shelled peas

6 asparagus stalks

1 cup pine nuts

Parmesan cheese (see p. 140)

1 teaspoon lemon juice

2 tablespoons cold-pressed extra-virgin olive oil

Himalayan salt to taste

Freshly milled pepper to taste

1 tablespoon mixed Italian herbs, fresh if possible

DIRECTIONS FOR ASPARAGUS

Wash the asparagus, and pat it dry. Break off the tough woodsy part, and compost it. Cut the asparagus in thin rounds, leaving the tips whole. The asparagus may be marinated and placed in a dehydrator to soften for 1 hour if desired.

DIRECTIONS FOR SAUCE

Place the pine nuts in a high-speed blender adding ½ cup water (add water slowly and not all at once). Add 1 teaspoon lemon juice, Italian herbs, olive oil salt, and pepper. Blend until smooth and thick. Add more water if necessary. Taste for seasonings, and adjust if necessary.

TO FINISH

Place the rice in a large mixing bowl. Toss in the peas and asparagus. Pour the pine nut cheese on top, and lightly mix it in. Warm the mixture in a dehydrator at 115° F or in an oven with the door left open at lowest temperature. Only warm to body temperature; do not overheat.

TO SERVE

Divide into bowls, and sprinkle with whole pine nuts and Parmesan cheese. Add chopped fresh basil leaves if desired.

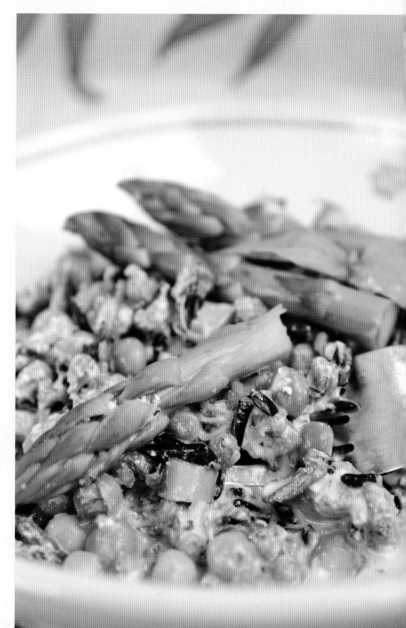

Dessert (Il Dolce)

Italian deserts are simply delicious. Bakeries and pastry shops are everywhere to tempt locals and tourists alike. There is no reason why us raw fooders can't enjoy some of these sweets, and I'm here to prove that the healthy version is as good as it gets.

Panna Cotta

Traditionally, panna cotta is made with cream, milk, sugar, and gelatin, but since we are not going in that direction, it was time for me to come up with a delicious raw, healthy version of this dish. What would the Italians say when they see I've conjured up new ways to alter their perfect classics? I'm not sure, but I have many Italian friends, and they like my raw dishes, so I hope they will continue to appreciate my effort.

1 cup cashews	½ cup sweetener of choice
1 teaspoon vanilla extract	½ cup Irish moss paste (see p. 46)
1 teaspoon hazelnut extract	5 tablespoons coconut oil
1 cup young Thai coconut meat	½ cup water if needed

DIRECTIONS

In a high-speed blender, grind the cashews and add the coconut meat, sweetener, vanilla, hazelnut extract, coconut oil, and Irish moss paste. Blend lightly, slowly increasing the speed and using a tamper to push down the mixture. Work the tamper around in a circle to keep the mixture moving. Add water slowly, if necessary, and keep the tamper moving. Stop for a few minutes so the blender doesn't overheat. The mixture should be smooth without coconut lumps. You might have to stop the blender a couple of times while mixing. Use as little liquid as possible to keep the mixture thick. If there are still small coconut pieces, place half of the mixture into a bowl, and mix half at a time in the blender until smooth.

Scoop into serving dishes, and chill in a refrigerator for 4–5 hours. Garnish with whole berries. In a blender, mix some berries with maple syrup and a touch of water, if necessary, to make a sauce for topping.

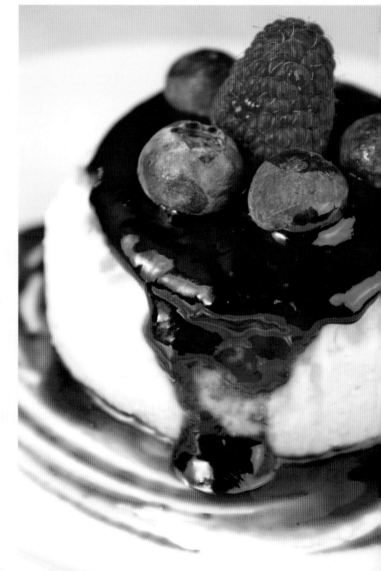

Tiramisu—Simply Raw

(8–10 small servings)

Traditional tiramisu contains raw eggs, ladyfingers, and mascarpone cheese. There was no way to exactly duplicate this recipe. Even though there are layers, I've made this desert as simple as possible. I believe you will be happy with this classic Italian dessert made the healthy way. I like using small cheesecake molds, the bottom of which pushes up and keeps a nice shape for one serving (they resemble cupcake pans except for the push-up bottom and straight sides).

LAYER 1: CAKE

1 cup pecans

6 Medjool dates

1 teaspoon coffee extract (see p. 66)

4 tablespoons cacao powder

1–2 teaspoons rum extract (see p. 66)

DIRECTIONS

Blend all ingredients in a food processor until they stick together when pinched between your fingers. Taste for sweetness and flavor, and adjust if necessary. Press the mixture into the molds.

LAYER 2: CREAM

1 cup cashews, soaked for 2–3 hours

1 cup young Thai coconut meat

2 teaspoons vanilla extract or scraped beans from 1 vanilla bean

⅓ cup maple syrup

5 tablespoons coconut oil, melted

Water as needed

DIRECTIONS

Grind the cashews to flour. In a high-speed blender, place the nuts, coconut meat, vanilla, and maple syrup, and blend until smooth. Add just enough water to keep the mixture moving. Pile cream on top of the cake layer, and tap the dish down lightly to set this layer. Refrigerate until set firm.

LAYER 3: TOPPING

You will be happy to know that this layer is only raw sifted cacao powder. Use enough to cover the top of the cream with a very light layer. Pour the cacao into a small hand strainer, and tap it as you move over the top of the molds.

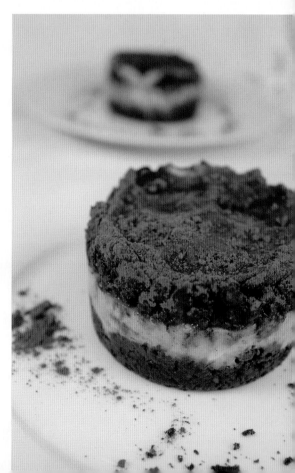

Pear Sorbetto

(4–6 servings)

5–6 pears, really ripe and
soft, skin removed

½ cup sucanat, ground
to a fine powder, or any
sweetener of choice

2½ cups water

1 tablespoon lemon juice

Pear extract: a drop is sometimes
helpful to enhance the flavor,
as pears can be unpredictable
(see p. 66)

DIRECTIONS

Blend all ingredients in a high-speed blender until completely smooth, adding more water if necessary. Taste for sweetness and lemon, adding more if necessary to your liking.

Pour into a flat dish, and place in a freezer. Whisk with a fork every half hour. The sorbet will be ready to eat in 2 or so hours. If you leave it overnight, let it sit out for 5 minutes, then place it in a blender and tamper it down to achieve a scoopable texture.

TO SERVE

Serve with a sprig of mint or basil on top.

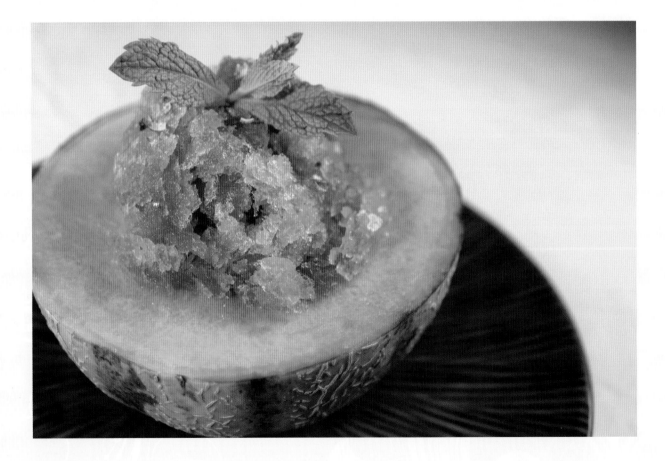

Beverages (Bevanda)

The Perfect Limonata

When life gives you lemons, make lemonade. A simple recipe sometimes needs the perfect balance of lemon juice, water, and sweetener. Once you learn this method, the guesswork is in the past.

What could be more refreshing on a hot summer day than ice-cold lemonade, or in Italy, limonata, which can be effervescent? We are going to give this lemonade/limonata an Italian twist by adding basil. The best-tasting lemonade is always made with simple syrup, which consists of water and sugar heated in a pan until the mixture thickens. It is stored in the refrigerator to use in cocktails and drinks. Our simple syrup will be made with stevia or xylitol because other sugars, like maple syrup or coconut crystals, will turn the lemonade brown. The amount of stevia drops can vary as some lemons are sweeter than others and our taste buds can be different. When I use Meyer lemons from our garden, I don't use much sweetener, as Meyer lemons are very sweet on their own. Did you know that most stevia powder contains lactose (milk)? Using liquid stevia works well for us vegans. If you don't mind brown lemonade, use maple syrup, coconut crystals, or sweetener of choice.

LIMONATA

1 cup lemon juice, freshly squeezed (Meyer lemon when possible)

1 cup simple syrup (see recipe below)

2–3 cups water, depending on desired taste

SIMPLE SYRUP

¼ cup basil leaves

1 cup water

1 teaspoon stevia, more or less, depending on personal taste

DIRECTIONS FOR SYRUP

Place all ingredients into a blender, and blend until smooth. Pour into a pitcher.

TO FINISH

Stir the lemon juice, simple syrup, and water together in a pitcher, and chill in a refrigerator.

TO SERVE

Place ice in glasses, pour in lemonade, and garnish with a sprig of basil and a lemon twist.

TIP { For a carbonated drink, add ½ cup San Pellegrino or bubbly water of choice. San Pellegrino is high in calcium and magnesium, and low in salt.

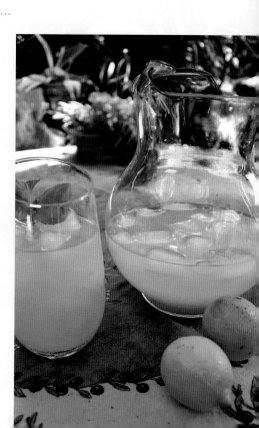

Virgin Italian Sunrise

Freshly-squeezed orange juice   Homemade grenadine

POMEGRANATE GRENADINE

Juice from 2 pomegranates (see instructions below) or juice from 2 cups dark cherries may also be used

Maple syrup, or sweetener of choice, to taste

DIRECTIONS FOR POMEGRANATE GRENADINE

To extract the seeds from a pomegranate, fill a large bowl with water. You will need to get both hands in the bowl. Place the pomegranate in the bowl, and cut it across its center. Pull the pomegranate apart, start breaking off a piece, and pull seeds out underwater gently with your fingers. The thin membrane will float to the top, and the seeds will sink to the bottom. Toss the outside skin out of the bowl as you proceed. Repeat with the second pomegranate. Slowly tip the bowl, and pour the water out. The membranes will float out. Any that are stuck at the bottom usually contain seeds. Use your fingers to loosen them when the majority of the water is out. Pour the balance, including the seeds, through a colander. Place the seeds in a mesh strainer, and press with the back of a spoon to release juice into a bowl. If you put seeds through your juicer or blender, the juice will be cloudy because of the white seeds. This method is fine for normal pomegranate juicing, but for this recipe I prefer pressing out the juice by hand.

DIRECTIONS FOR CHERRY GRENADINE

Pit the cherries, and run them through a juicer. Strain any pulp out.

TO ASSEMBLE DRINK

Pour the orange juice in a wine glass until three-fourth full. Take a tablespoonful of the grenadine, place the tip of the spoon against the glass, and slowly pour the liquid down the side. The grenadine will fall to the bottom. Repeat until one-third of the amount of grenadine appears on the bottom of the orange juice. Garnish with an orange rind curl made by using a potato peeler and stripping off a piece of orange peel. Scrap off some of the white under the part, and curl around a pencil or skewer.

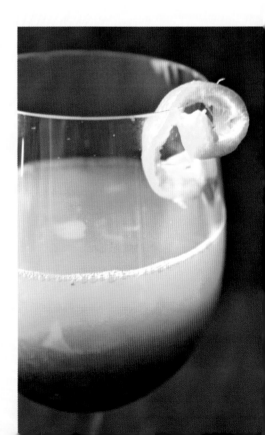

Simple Italian Drink

1½ cups dark grape juice

1 cup pomegranate juice

½ cup beet juice

½ cup coconut sugar or sweetener of choice

DIRECTIONS

Juice the grapes, pomegranates, and beets. Place them in a blender with the sweetener, and blend well. Serve chilled.

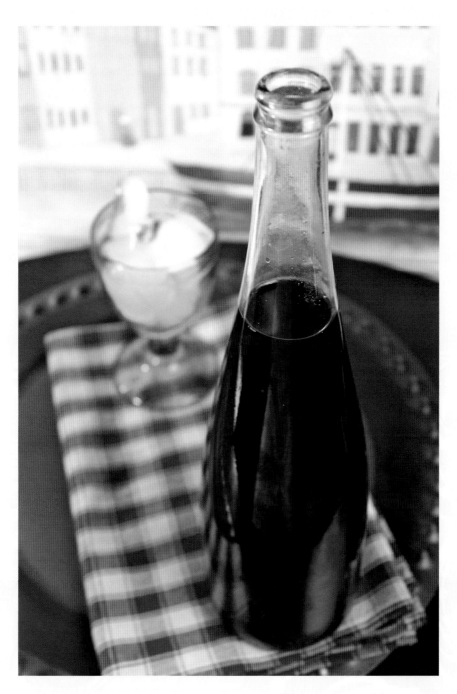

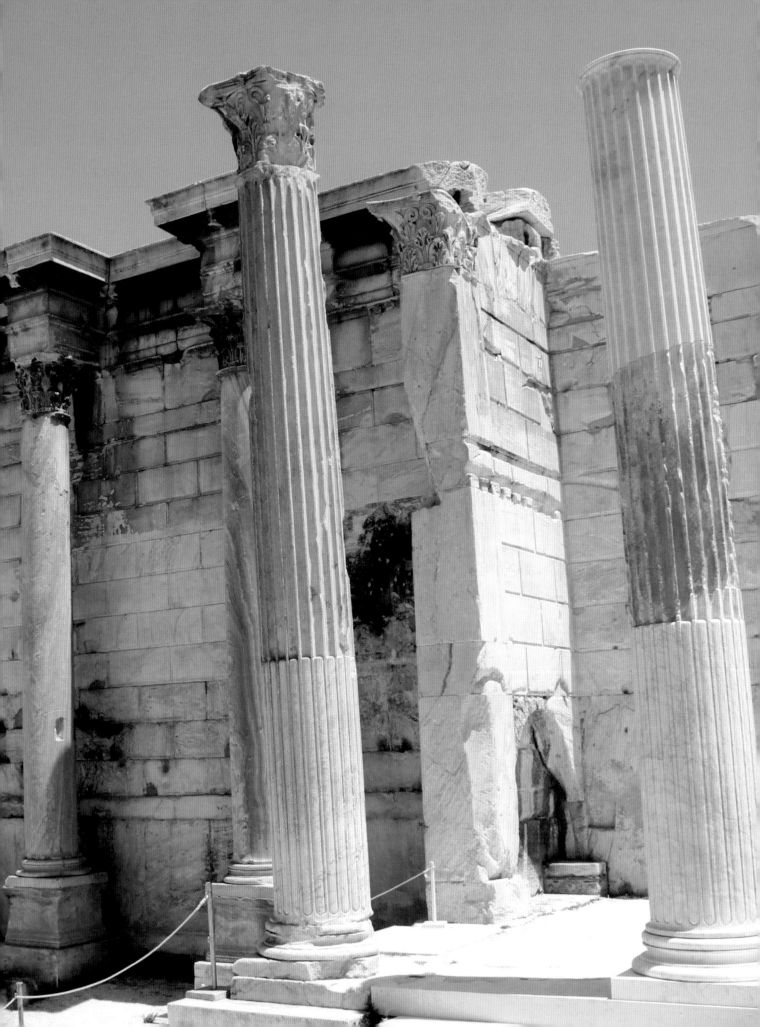

CHAPTER 15

·····················

RAW CUISINE—TASTE OF
GREECE

·····················

'd never been to Greece and was really looking forward to this trip. We started out in Athens, where I gave a talk to a packed house at Avocado for Life, a restaurant where we stopped almost every day to have our morning green drink. We ate some wonderful meals there, too. The owners, Eraj and Vivi, two of the sweetest people I've known, own a yoga studio across the street where Vivi teaches. The staff at Avocado for Life, including Harris and Vicky and a dedicated team, took great care of us. Avocado for Life primarily has a vegetarian/vegan menu and is adding more raw food regularly to its menu.

The Lalki (popular market) in Athens is a very large street market. Just about every village has a street market at least once a week. In a large town, you can find a market every day in a different neighborhood. Vendors encourage tasting their fruit or vegetables before you buy so they can prove theirs is the best. Along with all the beautiful colorful foods, we found just about everything and anything you might need for your household. It's always been difficult for me to resist local tableware when traveling, and I continually have to remind myself how heavy these items can be to carry home. More than once I found myself lugging an extra bag of breakables through the airport and onto the plane. As I held up a beautiful platter to examine, I saw Mike a few feet away give me a smile, and I knew exactly what he was thinking, that is, he would be the one doing the lifting to carry it back home, so I put it down and walked away.

There were crowds of people in Athens, and taking photographs was difficult. We squeezed in at a stall where we were told the herbs were gathered that morning in the mountains. Oregano, chamomile, spearmint, and sage were just a few of the fragrant smells. The array of fruit and vegetables piled high at each stand makes you realize how hard vendors work to bring their produce to the market. We also learned that at the end of the day prices drop on fresh fruits and vegetables, as they are either very ripe or the vendor hopes to haul as little home as possible. Several stalls did not sell their own produce but were middlemen for farmers. I tend to like buying directly from farmers who grow their own crops because I can feel their passion about what they are selling. There were many clothing stalls, and behind them you could find a van or a little cordoned off place where you could try something on. Yes, of course, I just had to try something on, not that I needed any more clothes on this trip, but it was just too tempting at four Euros a blouse.

What differentiates one market from the next in each country? I would have to say the people. Food looks much the same at most fresh street markets except for a few local specialties. But the energy of the people can be

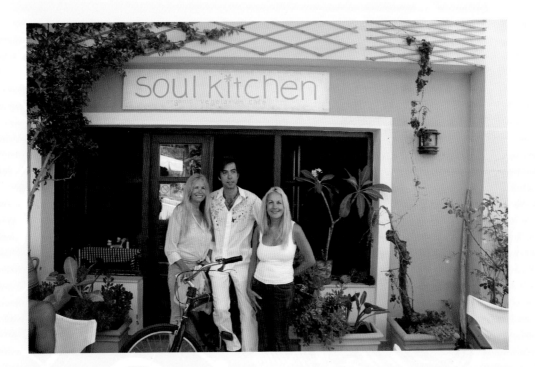

very different from country to country. You might say that if you've been to one street market in a foreign country, you've been to them all, but I personally don't feel that way. Maybe it's because I'm a foodie, maybe because I love discovering that one little thing that's different in each country's market, or maybe I'm just an adventurer at heart. I always look at each market as a new exciting experience, and you never know what you will learn when you are open to the unknown.

After several days touring Athens, we moved on to Crete and a town called Rethymnon. We met George Cassimedes, owner of Triopetra Yoga Retreat and Soul Kitchen, his vegetarian restaurant next door. George made us delicious green drinks each day we were there. He purchases his produce from a local organic farmers market. Every morning after yoga, the family-style outdoor tables were packed with hungry yoga students from around the world.

George took us to beautiful beaches and outdoor restaurants right on the water's edge that only locals knew about. He mentioned to me that there was a sadhu who lived in Rethymnon outside by a stream for the past twenty-three years. A sadhu is someone who has chosen to live apart from society in order to focus on his or her own spiritual practice. Such people are respected for their holiness and considered living embodiments of the divine.

George said we could visit him. One morning, we set out on the journey over narrow, bumpy dirt roads and down to the riverbank in the middle of a valley where the sadhu lived. If you didn't know exactly where he lived, you'd never know he was there. George crossed the stream alone and in a few minutes, he reappeared and motioned for me to come over. I crossed the shallow rocky stream and there, in his cave-like living quarters under a tree and hidden from view, was the eighty-year-old sadhu. He motioned for me to come in and sit down. I was expecting him to be Indian, but his light blue eyes said something different; he was an American.

I learned that he took the vow of renunciation and left the material world behind in 1968. He spent many years in India with his guru, acquiring the necessary experiences before moving on. He taught meditation in India for years before heading to Greece. I spent a good half hour with him, and he was very welcoming and kind. He ate one meal a day, was very thin, and had long matted white hair. His sleeping quarters were a thin mattress with a tarp underneath to keep his bed dry. There was a mosquito net over the bed, lots of books, and even a battery-operated clock. He was wearing only a loincloth, and he was sitting in an old wooden meditation seat. He was clean, and so was his organized environment. His bathing towel was hanging on a branch, drying. Locals like George brought him food and looked in on him. During the winter months, he moved to the other side of the stream, where he could be protected from the cold.

I was quite comfortable sitting on a yellow blanket next to him as we spoke. To both our surprise, we knew of each other's gurus and found we had acquaintances in common from our former spiritual days. We talked about many things past and present. I'm still in disbelief that under a tree, on a stream in Rethymnon, Greece, I meet a holy man with whom I could sit and have a conversation like he was a long-lost friend. This is one experience I'll certainly never forget.

I was surprised to be recognized in a restaurant one evening in Rethymonon by a couple visiting from Lithuania, Dalius and Egle Regelskis. They didn't want to approach me at dinner, so they e-mailed me that evening to let me know they saw me. We met the next day at George's restaurant for green drinks. Egle is a well-known swing dancer, and Dalius is an architect. They are primarily raw foodists, have a copy of *Live Raw*, and occasionally post recipes they've made from my book on my Facebook page. They are very beautiful and sweet people.

One can find paradise in Greece with its 3,000 islands to choose from to visit. Hopefully, this will not be my last visit to Greece as there is so much to experience, including beaches, archaeological sites, museums, wonderful people, and Greek salads.

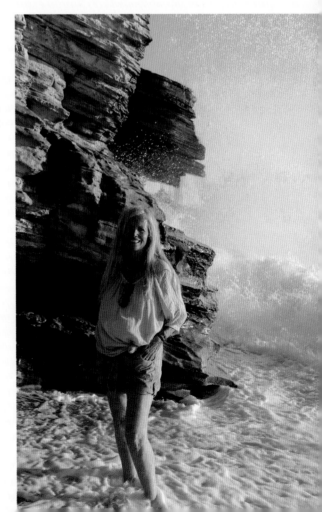

greek herbs and spices

Greek food is not spicy, but very flavorful. Herbs are grown everywhere throughout Greece, and the fragrance in the air cannot be avoided. One can find herbs and spices growing on almost every kitchen windowsill and wild all over the mountainsides. Salt is the most popular way to bring the flavors out of the food, and salt from the sea is of the highest quality and used on every table. Pepper is also on every table, adding flavor and a tiny bit of spice. If I had to pick one spice that defines Greek food, I would choose oregano. Other common herbs include marjoram, sage, thyme, basil, cloves, rosemary, mint, fennel, saffron, paprika, allspice, nutmeg, dill, parsley, coriander, bay leaves, parsley, cumin, cinnamon, anise, cardamom, and coriander. You can combine a pinch or so of several herbs to make a blend. The oregano on the island of Crete is some of the best I've ever tasted, and the mountain herb tea is addictive.

Kalí Órexi (Enjoy Your Meal)

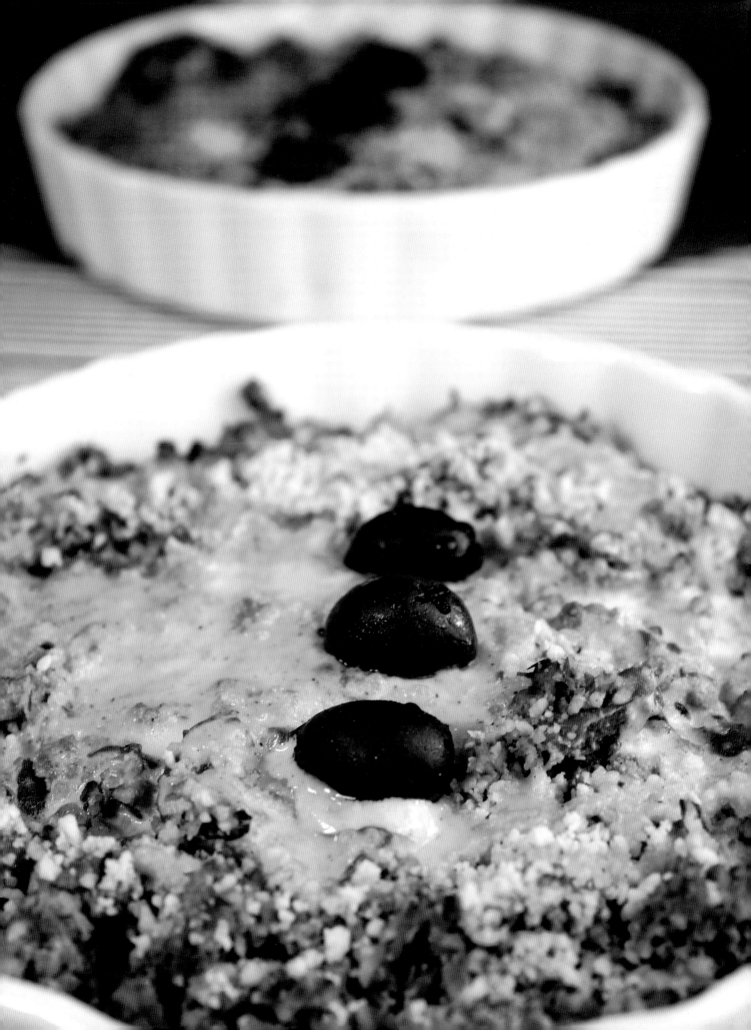

Breakfast (Proinó)

Greeks are not big on breakfast. Only in tourist hotels can you find the usual American breakfast fare.

The green drink lives on in Greece with those who are health conscious. I was able to find delicious morning green drinks in both Athens and Crete.

Greek Green Drink with Lemon Verbena Tea, Coconut Yogurt, Clementines, and Greens

- 2 handfuls dark leafy greens of your choice
- 2 clementines, peeled and seeded (oranges my be substituted)
- ½ cup coconut yogurt, or more if desired (see p. 160)
- 2 cups lemon verbena tea (see directions below)

DIRECTIONS

Verbena is known for it stimulating effect on the digestive tract, aiding in digestion. Verbena calms the nerves, and some say it helps with weight loss, fatigue, and autoimmune diseases. To make the tea, boil water, place a tea bag in a cup or teapot and let steep 15 minutes. When cool, pour into a blender. Add the remaining ingredients, and blend until smooth.

Shredded Apple, Almond Milk, and Fruit

(2 servings)

This simple breakfast is easy and satisfying.

- 2 apples, shredded
- 1 tablespoon lemon juice
- 1 cup almond or cashew milk reserved for serving (see p. 65)
- 1 small handful almonds, chopped
- 3 tablespoons coconut yogurt (optional; see p. 160)
- 3 chopped dates or ¼ cup raisins
- 1 banana, thinly sliced
- Maple syrup to taste or honey for those who prefer it and are not vegan (honey is very popular in Greece)

DIRECTIONS

Shred the apples with an attachment of a food processor or with a grater, and mix with lemon juice. Lightly toss in the remaining ingredients, and serve in a beautiful bowl.

TO SERVE

Add fruit on top, a dollop of coconut yogurt, chilled almond milk, amount to your liking, and a drizzle of sweetener. This mixture can be slightly warmed in cold days.

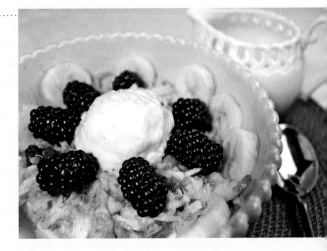

TIP Add cinnamon or any fruit or berries in season.

Pear and Cheese Turnover

(approx. 24 pieces; recipe may be cut in half)

DOUGH

2 cups almond pulp (see p. 65)

2 cups coconut meat

4 Medjool dates, soaked

2–3 tablespoons maple syrup or sweetener of choice

½ cup flax meal

½ cup psyllium meal (ground fine in coffee mill or spice grinder)

Himalayan salt to taste

¾ cup water

DIRECTIONS

Place the coconut meat, water, dates, salt, and maple syrup in a high-speed blender, and blend until smooth. Place the pulp, flax, and psyllium in a mixing bowl, and add the coconut mixture. Mix well with a spatula to incorporated the ingredients.

Filling

2 pears, thinly sliced on mandolin slicer (apples may also be used)

½ cup feta cheese (see p. 168)

1 teaspoon coconut sugar

1 teaspoon cinnamon

Blend cinnamon and sugar together.

TO ASSEMBLE

With a small pastry scooper or tablespoon, proportion the dough onto a nonstick dehydrator sheet. Flatten each portion into 3-inch rounds, approximately ⅛-inch thick. Place 2 pear slices folded over on one side of the dough, and spread ½ teaspoon cheese over the pears. Sprinkle with the cinnamon-sugar mixture. Lift the unfilled end with a large knife or pastry spatula, and fold over the filling. Crimp the edges closed by pressing down with a fork. Continue filling until all dough is used. Dehydrate for 2 hours at 110–115° F. Remove to mesh sheets, and dehydrate for 2–3 hours until dry. Turnovers will have a light outside crust and a soft center. The pieces are delicious served warm or at room temperature.

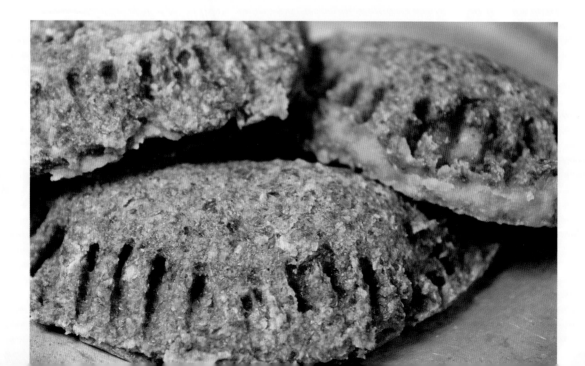

Orange Slices with Coconut Yogurt

(2 servings)

Breakfast in Greece is simple and just a quick way to start the day. I'm including this dish to give you an idea how easy and satisfying a simple meal can be. Any fruit may be used, but juiced oranges pack lots of vitamin C.

2 oranges

1 cup coconut yogurt

2 tablespoons maple syrup or sweetener of choice

DIRECTIONS

Peel and slice the oranges in thick rounds, removing the white part. Arrange the slices on a plate, and place a scoop of yogurt on each slice. Drizzle with a sweetener of choice.

COCONUT YOGURT

4 cups young Thai coconut meat

1 cup coconut water

2 capsules probiotics (open capsules) or 1 teaspoon powdered probiotics

DIRECTIONS

Place the coconut meat and probiotics in a high-speed blender. Add just enough coconut water to make a thick and very smooth mixture. Use a tamper and keep tamping down to keep the mixture moving, adding coconut water as needed. Transfer from the blender into a bowl or yogurt maker. Cover and keep in a very warm place overnight. I use a Donvier electric yogurt maker with eight small containers, which keeps the temperature at 90° F for 9 hours, or you could place the mixture in a dehydrator at 90° F for 8–9 hours. If neither a yogurt maker nor a dehydrator is available, pour the yogurt mixture in a mason jar, and place a cheesecloth or paper towel on top. Let the mixture sit in a warm place for 6 hours. Store in a refrigerator to firm up.

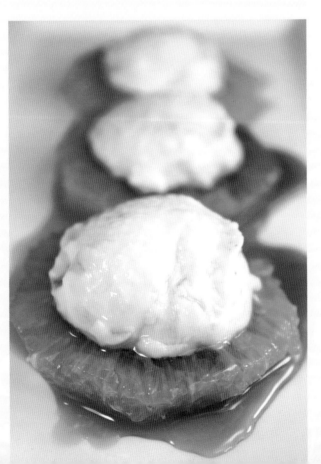

Lunch (Ariston)

Zucchini Falafel with Dill Cucumber Sauce

(4 servings)

FALAFEL

2 cups zucchini, shredded

1 cup sunflower seeds, finely ground

1 cup pumpkin seeds, finely ground

¼ cup onion, finely chopped, or ¼ cup shallot, finely chopped

1–2 cloves garlic, crushed

1 tablespoon lemon juice

Himalayan salt to taste

Freshly milled pepper to taste

½ teaspoon oregano

½ teaspoon coriander

½ teaspoon marjoram

DIRECTIONS

Shred the zucchini in a food processor until very fine. Grind the sunflower seeds in a spice mill or high-powered blender until fine. Grind the pumpkin seeds in a spice mill or high-powered blender until fine. Place the zucchini and both seeds in a mixing bowl, and add the chopped onion, crushed garlic, lemon juice, salt, pepper, and herbs. Mix well, using the back of a spatula to incorporate the ingredients. Roll the mixture into small balls, place on the mesh screen of a dehydrator tray, and dehydrate at 110° F for 10–15 hours. Leave to dehydrate until the outside forms a crust and the middle is slightly soft. Moisture varies with zucchini, so dehydrate until the balls are slightly firm.

DILL CUCUMBER SAUCE

1 cup coconut yogurt (see p. 160)

1 clove garlic, crushed

1 scallion, finely chopped

½ teaspoon oregano, finely chopped

1 teaspoon mint, finely chopped

1–2 teaspoons dill, finely chopped

1 cup English cucumber, peeled, seeded, and finely chopped or grated

Himalayan salt to taste

Freshly milled pepper to taste

DIRECTIONS

Wrap the chopped cumbers in a kitchen towel or cheesecloth, and squeeze out the liquid. Place all ingredients in a mixing bowl, and toss well. Taste for seasonings, and adjust if necessary. Refrigerate. The sauce is best made ahead so that the yogurt can absorb all the herb flavors. Add water, if necessary, to make a smooth sauce.

TO SERVE

Place each falafel on a lettuce leaf, cover with yogurt sauce, and add some chopped onions. Falafels are also delicious on pita bread (see p. 166).

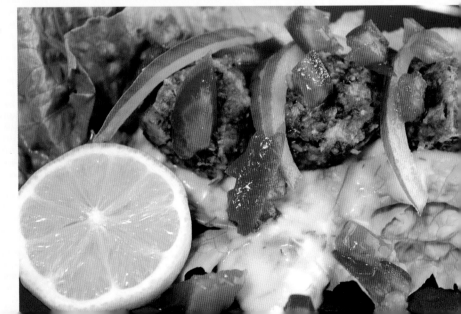

Kale Tabouleh Salad

(4 servings)

1 bunch kale, destemmed, washed, dried, and finely cut into small ribbons

1 bunch parsley, finely chopped

1 cup cucumber, peeled, seeded, and diced

¼ cup mint leaves, chopped

2 scallions, finely chopped

1 cup sprouted wild rice or hemp seeds

Dressing

1–2 cloves garlic, crushed

4 tablespoons lemon juice

1 tablespoon shallot, finely chopped

⅔ cup good-quality extra-virgin olive oil

1 teaspoon oregano, fresh if possible

Himalayan salt to taste

Freshly milled pepper to taste

DIRECTIONS

Place the salad ingredients in a small bowl, reserving the olive oil. Mix the ingredients, and slowly whisk in the olive oil a little at a time. Taste for seasonings, and adjust if necessary. A tiny drop of sweetener may be added.

Topping

Cut the cherry tomatoes in half, and marinate in the crushed garlic, olive oil, and salt.

TO SERVE

In a large salad bowl, massage the kale leaves with a drop or two of olive oil until softened. Add the remaining salad ingredients to the bowl, and lightly toss to combine. Pour the salad dressing on top, and toss well.

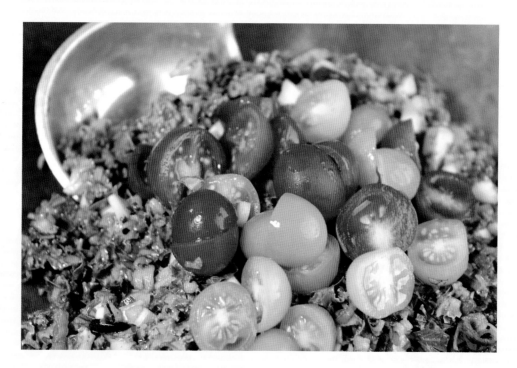

Classic Greek Salad

We wondered if Greek salad in Greece would just be called salad, but most menus called it Greek salad whereas smaller, nontourist places called it Village Salata. Including this very simple and delicious salad is a must. Use the best ingredients you can find. Red ripe tomatoes, firm cucumbers, and sweet onions are all the ingredients you need (although in America most Greek salads include lettuce). Feel free to include some if you wish, but I find this salad perfect the way the Greeks serve it. During summer, this salad is found everywhere in Greece, but in spring and winter salads consist of cabbage and carrots or cabbage and lettuce.

SALAD

(2 servings)

1 English cucumber, peeled and thickly sliced

2 tomatoes, cut into thick slices or chunks

Red onion, thinly sliced, amount of your choice

Black kalamata olives, raw if possible

Feta cheese (see p. 168), amount of your choice

Dressing

2–3 cloves garlic, crushed

1 tablespoon lemon juice

1 teaspoon apple cider vinegar

6 tablespoons extra-virgin olive oil

1 teaspoon fresh Greek oregano or ½ teaspoon dried

Himalayan salt to taste

Freshly milled pepper to taste

DIRECTIONS

Chill the salad ingredients while you make the dressing. Place all dressing ingredients in a large salad bowl, reserving the olive oil. Whisk the dressing ingredients, and slowly add oil, whisking continuously until the dressing is creamy. Taste for seasonings, and add more of anything you feel necessary. Place the salad mixture in bowl, add the dressing, and toss until all leaves are coated. Serve on a chilled plate or bowl.

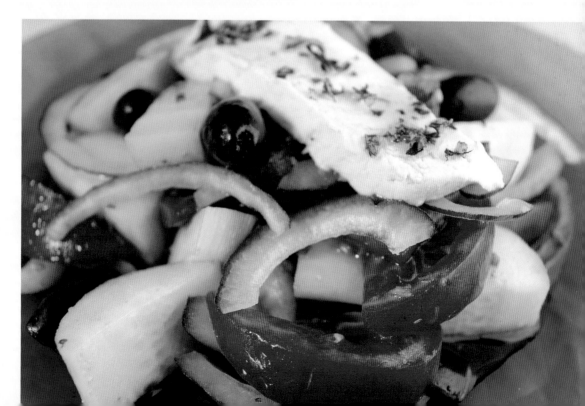

Dinner (Deipnon)

Eggplant Moussaka

(4 servings)

My daughter Mia inspired this dish when she told me that all she ate on her trip to Greece many years ago was Greek salad and moussaka. I thought she would enjoy this raw version of moussaka since her eating habits have changed. There are several steps to making raw moussaka, but not many more than in the traditional recipe.

1 eggplant, peeled and cut into ½-inch thick rounds (mandolin slicer works well)

½ cup olive oil

¼ cup gluten-free tamari

1 cup cashew béchamel sauce

2 cups sprouted rice (see p. 44)

½ cup cashew Parmesan cheese, grated

1 cup tomato sauce

PART 1: EGGPLANT PREPARATION

Peel the eggplants, and slice into ½-inch slices. Mix ½ cup olive oil and ¼ cup gluten-free tamari. Place the eggplant in a shallow baking dish, and marinate the slices. Add more oil and tamari if necessary to coat pieces. Place the eggplant slices on the mesh screen of a dehydrator tray, and dehydrate at 110°F for 2 hours. Turn the slices over halfway through the dehydration process.

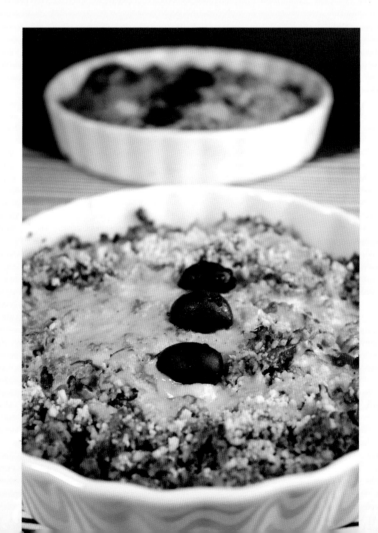

PART 2: SPROUTED RICE MIXTURE PREPARATION

2 cups sprouted wild rice (see p. 44)

1 cup walnuts

2 cloves garlic, crushed

¼ cup sweet onion, finely chopped

½ teaspoon cinnamon, ground

¼ teaspoon allspice, ground

1 tablespoon Greek herbs mix (see p. 52)

2 large tomatoes, coarsely chopped

1 teaspoon maple syrup or sweetener of choice

Himalayan salt to taste

Freshly milled pepper to taste

DIRECTIONS

Place 1 cup walnuts in a food processor, and pulse chop 2–3 times. Add the drained rice, and pulse chop again 4–5 times. Transfer to a bowl. Add the remaining ingredients, blending well. Blend the sun-dried tomatoes and chopped tomatoes in a food processor until chunky but incorporated. Add a little water a tablespoon at a time, if necessary, but keep the mixture thick and chunky. Add the tomatoes to the rice mixture. Add sweetener, cinnamon, allspice, salt, and Italian herbs, and blend well.

PART 3: WHITE SAUCE PREPARATION

1 cup cashews

1 cup water or almond milk

½ teaspoon nutmeg, ground

⅛ teaspoon cinnamon

2 tablespoons nutritional yeast

Himalayan salt to taste

DIRECTIONS

Blend the ingredients in a high-speed blender until smooth. Add Himalayan salt to taste.

PART 4: TOMATO SAUCE PREPARATION

2 large tomatoes, seeded

1 clove garlic

Himalayan salt to taste

DIRECTIONS

Place the ingredients in a food processor, and pulse chop until the pieces are broken up.

PART 5: PARMESAN CHEESE PREPARATION

(see p. 140)

TO ASSEMBLE

Rub olive oil on the bottom of a baking dish that will fit in your dehydrator. Four individual dishes may also be used. Put a small amount of tomato sauce on the bottom of the dish. Cut the eggplant into bite-size pieces, and place a layer on top of the sauce. Add a layer of the sprouted rice mixture. Sprinkle Parmesan cheese on top. Repeat the layers. Pour cashew béchamel sauce over the top, and gently tap the dish down to settle the sauce. Place the dish on a dehydrator tray, and dehydrate 1–2 hours at 110° F until warmed. If you don't have a dehydrator, you can use your oven at the lowest temperature with the door ajar. Be careful not to cook the ingredients; keep this dish raw. Heat the ingredients to body temperature.

TO SERVE

If using a large baking dish, scoop out a portion with a serving spoon onto individual dishes.

Pita Wrapped Gyro with Dill Cucumber Sauce

(4–5 servings)

Pita

1¾ cups oat groats	1 cup water
1 teaspoon Himalayan salt	

DIRECTIONS

Grind the groats to flour in a high-speed blender or spice grinder (see p. 44). Add 1 cup water, and blend to combine. Place the dough in a bowl, and knead a few times. Flatten out on a nonstick dehydrator tray, pressing with fingers to make approximately 4–5 five-inch rounds. The dough will be a little sticky, but just keep working to flatten it out. Dehydrate for 15–20 minutes at 115° F. After 15 minutes, flip the nonstick sheet over onto a mesh sheet. Handle gently, using a large chopping knife to help peel the pita off the sheet and loosen the soft sticky spots. Dehydrate for another 15–20 minutes on the mesh screen. Press on the thickest part of the pita to test doneness. The pita should be slightly soft in the center. Do not overdehydrate, but make sure it is done. Pitas are best warm but store well in a refrigerator. To store, wrap the pita in a paper towel, and place it in a Ziploc bag. The pita will soften as it sits, and it can be put back in the dehydrator to warm up.

Mushroom Filling

2 large portobello mushrooms	Himalayan salt to taste
⅛ teaspoon each cumin, curry, savory, paprika, oregano, and thyme	Freshly milled pepper to taste
	3 tablespoons gluten-free tamari
2 large cloves garlic, crushed	3 tablespoons olive oil

DIRECTIONS

Wipe the mushrooms with a damp paper towel. Remove the stems and gills from the underside by using a teaspoon or melon baller. Cut off the thinner rim that curves in, leaving a solid piece of mushroom. Slice the mushrooms thinly with a sharp knife. Marinate the pieces in spices, tamari, and olive oil for 10 minutes. Place on a dehydrator sheet, and dehydrate at 110° F for 1 hour.

Pita Filling

Lettuce or spinach	¼ red onion, thinly sliced
2 tomatoes, seeded, sliced in small wedges	Dill cucumber sauce (see p. 161)

TO ASSEMBLE

Spread the yogurt sauce on the pita, place lettuce or spinach on top, then layer with mushrooms, tomatoes, and onions. Roll at an angle with the larger opening at one end, or fold over in half.

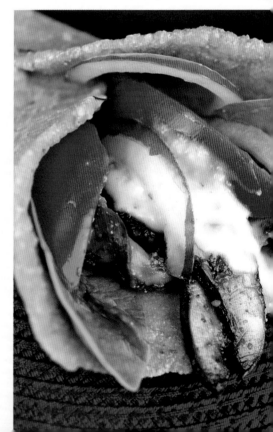

Stuffed Tomatoes and Zucchini with Sprouted Wild Rice and Feta Cheese

(4 servings)

2 zucchinis, cut in half lengthwise, centers hollowed out

4 medium-size tomatoes, tops cut off, centers gently hollowed out

DIRECTIONS

Rub the zucchinis and tomatoes with olive oil. Place them in a baking dish with a little water on the bottom, and dehydrate for 1 hour at 115° F to soften.

Filling

1½ cups sprouted wild rice (see p. 44)

1 cup raw feta cheese (see recipe that follows)

½ cup onion, finely chopped

DIRECTIONS

Mix the rice, cheese, and onion together in a small bowl.

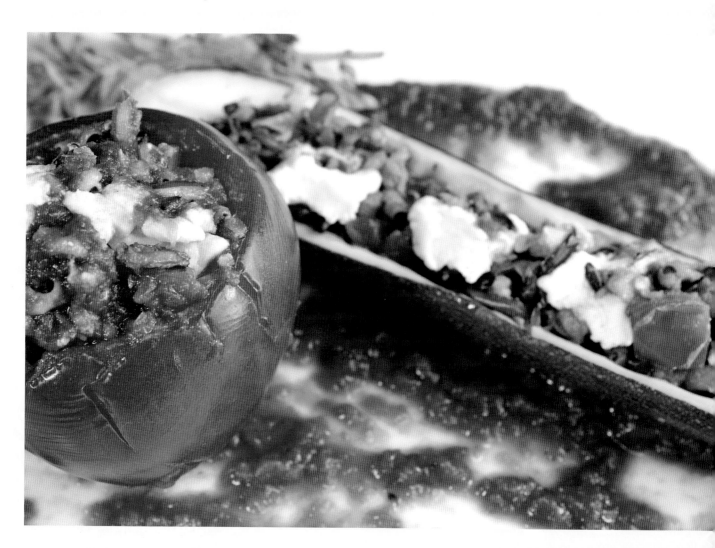

Sauce

- 1 small garlic clove, crushed
- ½ cup sun-dried tomatoes, soaked until soft
- 2 large red ripe tomatoes, seeded and coarsely chopped
- ½ teaspoon dried oregano or 1 tablespoon fresh, finely chopped
- ½ teaspoon dried thyme or 1 tablespoon fresh, finely chopped
- Himalayan salt to taste
- Freshly milled pepper to taste
- ½ cup best you can buy extra-virgin olive oil
- 1 tablespoon lemon juice or apple cider vinegar
- Dash of sweetener if necessary to smooth out taste

DIRECTIONS

Combine all sauce ingredients in a high-speed blender until smooth and add to the rice mixture, reserving some for topping. Taste for seasonings, and adjust if necessary. With a small spoon, fill the tomato and zucchini cavities. Dehydrate in a glass baking dish with a little water on the bottom for 1–3 hours to warm. Serve with a tomato sauce topping.

Feta Cheese

This recipe will make more than you need for stuffing tomatoes, but you might want to have extra on hand for salads or to eat with raw crackers. You can also cut this recipe in half if you prefer no leftovers.

- 2 cups cashews, almonds, or macadamia nuts, soaked 2 hours (if using almonds, soak overnight and remove skins)
- 1 cup water
- the powder from 1 probiotic capsule
- Himalayan sea salt to taste, approximately 1 teaspoon or more

DIRECTIONS

Place the drained nuts into a high-speed blender, slowly adding water as needed to arrive at a smooth creamy texture. Add salt a little at a time, and taste. Scrape the mixture into a cheesecloth that is placed in a strainer and set over a bowl. Fold the cloth over the cheese, and put a weight on top, which will help extract any extra liquid. Let the cheese ferment for 12–48 hours in a dark place on the kitchen counter. Taste for desired tartness. Remove from the strainer. If desired, drop small dollops of cheese on a nonstick dehydrator tray, and dehydrate for 5 hours at 115° F, or use as is. After stuffing the tomatoes and zucchinis, the remainder of cheese may be stored in an airtight container in a refrigerator for a week.

Desserts (Érimos)
Baklava

(approx. 12 rounds)

Filo Dough

1½ cups cashews, soaked 3–4 hours

2 tablespoons lemon juice

2 tablespoons maple syrup or sweetener of choice

1 tablespoon vanilla extract

½ cup water

DIRECTIONS

Place all ingredients in a high-speed blender, and blend until completely smooth. Divide the mixture onto 2 nonstick dehydrator sheets, and tap the trays on the kitchen counter to help spread the mixture over the entire sheet. Use a pastry spatula to spread very thin. Dehydrate at 115° F for 5–6 hours or until a piece can be removed from the sheet. The piece will resemble fruit leather. Do not overdry, as the sheets must be flexible to roll in the filling. The center usually dries last, and the ends could get too dry. If the ends start drying, peel up around the loose edges, and when reaching the center soft spot, place the tray with a mesh screen on top of a nonstick sheet, and flip over. Using a large sharp knife, help peel away the sheet from the baklava. Dry a little longer, checking to be sure the sheets are still pliable.

Filling

1½ cups pistachios

½ cup walnuts

¼ teaspoon clove powder

⅛ teaspoon cinnamon

¼ teaspoon cardamom powder

Pinch of salt

½ tablespoon vanilla extract

1–2 tablespoons maple syrup or sweetener of choice

DIRECTIONS

Pulse chop all ingredients in a food processor, except the sweetener. Do not overprocess the nuts into a powder, just into small chunks. Place into a bowl, and add the sweetener so the mixture sticks together. Store in a refrigerator until ready to use.

TO ASSEMBLE

When the dough is dry, carefully cut it with kitchen scissors into 3-inch strips. Brush with maple syrup, and place a generous spoonful of filling about 2 inches from the end. Fold the 2-inch piece over the filling, and begin to roll to the end. Cut each piece in half with a sharp knife, and brush the open ends with maple syrup. Layers can also be made by cutting the dough into triangles, but I find the rolls easier to eat.

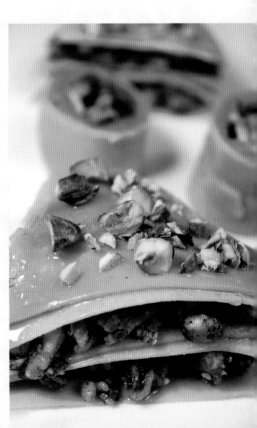

Greek Rice Pudding (ree-ZOH-ghah-loh)

(2 servings)

- 1 cup sprouted wild rice (see p. 44)
- 4 tablespoons chia seeds
- 2 cups nut milk (see p. 65)

- ½ teaspoon cinnamon
- 4 tablespoons maple syrup or sweetener of choice to taste

DIRECTIONS

Pour the nut milk in a bowl, and add the chia seeds. Whisk to combine. Whisk again in 10 minutes to break up any lumps. Add the rice, cinnamon, and sweetener, and whisk well. Repeat again in 10 minutes. When the mixture thickens, refrigerate to firm up and chill. A wire whisk or electric hand beater works well for smoothing out any lumps.

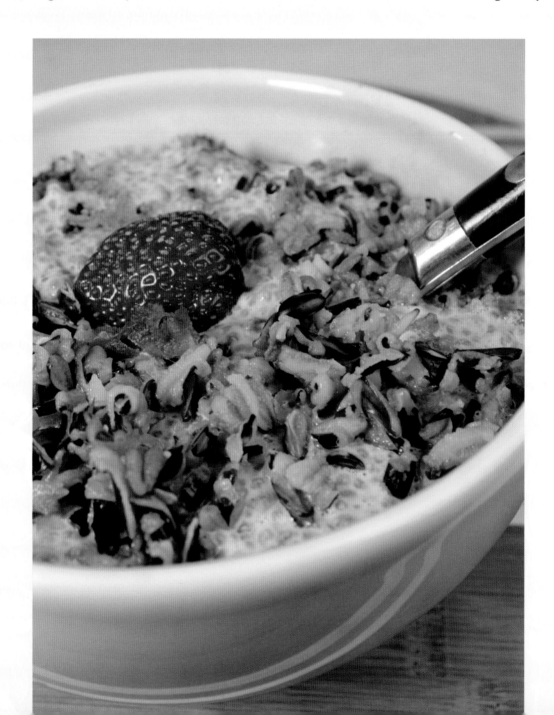

Date Pie

(6–8 servings)

Crust

½ cup sesame seeds	2 Medjool dates, softened in water
½ cup hemp seeds	Pinch of salt

DIRECTIONS

Pulse chop the ingredients in a food processor until combined. Line a glass pie pan with plastic wrap, or use 2 smaller pans with removable bottoms. Press the mixture onto the pan to form crust.

Filling

1 cup Medjool dates	½ cup cashews
½ cup almonds	10 Medjool dates, cut into halves and reserve for center layer

DIRECTIONS

Place the 1 cup dates, almonds, and cashews in a food processor. Pulse chop until the mixture forms a ball.
To assemble: Layer the cut dates on top of the crust, take a small amount of chopped filling, and press over the top of halved dates. Continue layering until the entire mixture is used.

TIP { This dish is delicious served warm. Place in a dehydrator until warmed, or in an oven at the lowest temperature for 10–15 minutes. Make a cashew cream topping (see p. [**]). A small piece goes a long way.

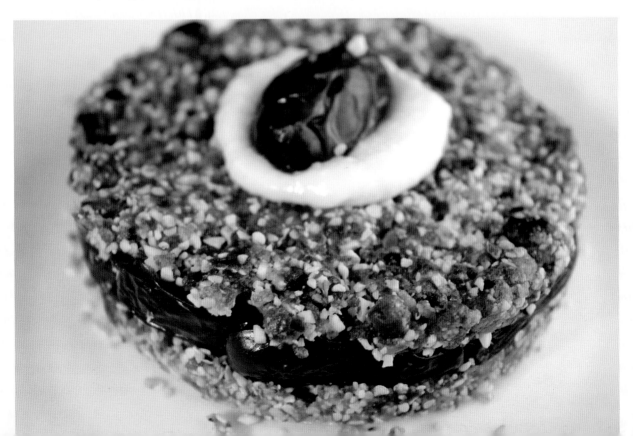

Beverages (Rofimata) (nonalcholic drinks)

Frappe can be several things: a liqueur poured over shaved ice, a frothy thick milkshake, or a frozen dessert with a mushy consistency. Our frappe recipe is a combination of milkshake and frozen dessert.

Frothy Thick Frappe

1 teaspoon coffee extract

1 cup water

1 cup almond or cashew milk

5 teaspoons cacao syrup

1 cup crushed ice

Extra sweetener of your choice to taste

DIRECTION

Dissolve the coffee extract in the water, and freeze in ice cube trays.

Cacao Syrup

½ cup maple syrup or liquid sweetener of choice

3 tablespoons cacao powder

1 tablespoon coconut oil, melted

1 tablespoon cacao butter, melted

Seeds from ½ vanilla bean or ½ teaspoon vanilla extract

2 teaspoons lucuma or mesquite powder

DIRECTION

Place the cacao powder, lucuma or mesquite, vanilla, and sweetener in a high-speed blender. Turn the blender on low speed. While the blender is running, add the melted coconut oil and cacao butter. The mixture can be stored in a refrigerator in a sealed container and softened by setting in a container of warm water.

DIRECTIONS

In a high-speed blender, place the milk, cacao syrup, and coffee ice cubes, and process until smooth. Add the crushed ice, and blend on low for a few seconds. Pour into chilled glasses, and drizzle cacao syrup on top.

Frosted Lime Drink

1 cup water

2 limes, juiced

Sweetener of choice to taste

DIRECTIONS

Blend all ingredients together, and pour into ice cube trays.

Mint Syrup

½ cup maple syrup, or sweetener of choice

4 mint leaves

Juice from 6 limes, approx. ¾ cup

DIRECTIONS

Crush the mint leaves in the sweetener, and set aside. Pour the lime juice, syrup, and 2 cups water in a high-speed blender. Blend, and add frozen lime cubes. Blend on low to break up the cubes and make the lime juice frothy.

TIP { To frost a glass, wet it and place it in a freezer. Once it's nicely frosted, remove from the freezer, moisten the rim with a slice of lime or lemon, and dip it into coconut sugar. Carbonated water may be added instead of flat water. If adding carbonated water, do not blend but just add to the glass with lime mixture.

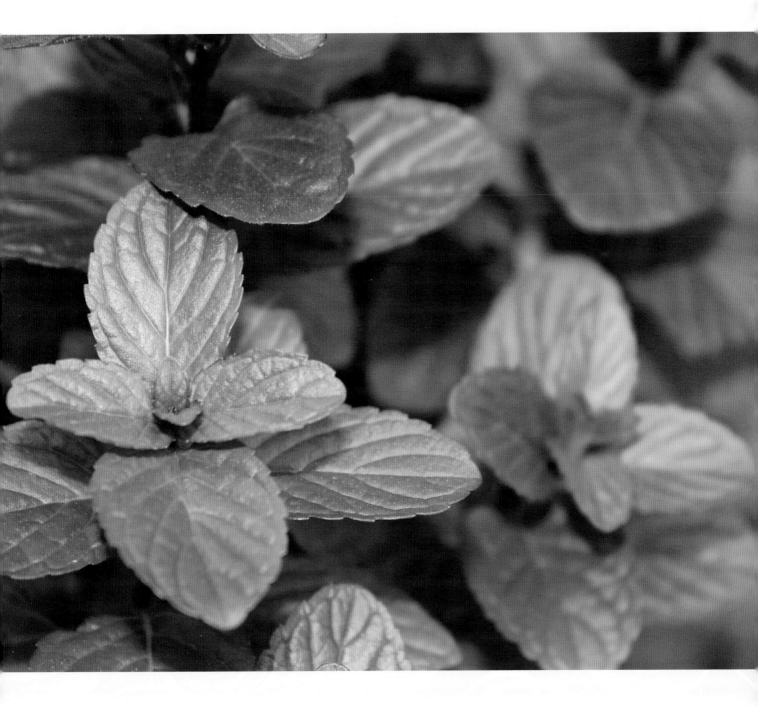

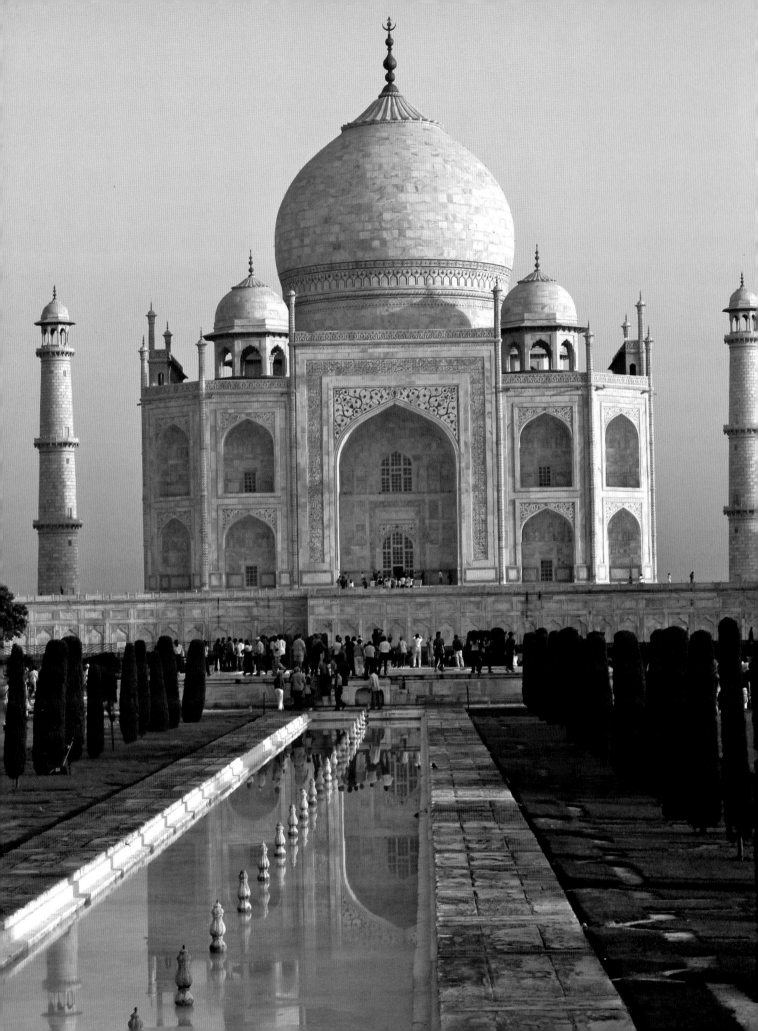

CHAPTER 16

. . . .

RAW CUISINE—TASTE OF

INDIA

. . . .

My first trip to India was to study in my guru's ashram in Ganispuri. My last trip to India was in 1986, for my friend Rakesh's wedding. It was the most thrilling wedding I've ever attended. The colors, tents, flowers, and beautiful bride Deepti in her red and gold sari made a picture in my mind to last a lifetime.

As I mentioned earlier, my daughter Lisa joined us on our passage to India. This was her first trip to India, and we all flew in together from Los Angeles. After a very long flight, my dear friend Rakesh, whom I call my Indian son, picked us up at the airport. We were taken to his lovely home with marble elephants and giant cement goddess statues leading to the front doorway. It was 2 AM, and we were tired from the long trip, but we stayed up and chatted. The next morning, we awoke to the smell of cinnamon and cardamom, as two small glasses of chai were placed on the side table of our bed.

I realized that eating raw in India would be more than a challenge. That morning for breakfast, I had fruit and a little rice, and enjoyed my chai. I was surprised to find that both Rakesh and his brother Krishna drank a green drink of their own concoction every morning. I've included the drink in this chapter, but be forewarned: It's not for the faint of heart. Rakesh downs his drink like a shot of whisky, while I sip mine. The drink is very bitter, but somehow I managed to enjoy it, well, sort of. I guess I was just happy to have a green drink. I could feel its potency running through my veins and later in my stomach.

After breakfast, Krishna came to see us with his wife, Madhu, an artist of beautiful spiritual paintings, and daughter Smriti, a jewelry designer. Smriti purchased my book when it first came out and brought it to her parents' home to show them a new way to eat healthfully. Her father took one look at the book and said, "I know Mimi, and we have been friends for years. She's our American mum."

I've known Rakesh and his brother Krishna since the early eighties when I met them at our guru's ashram in Los Angeles. We became very close over the years. We had not seen each other for a while, and he had no idea I had written a book. For his daughter Smriti to show up with it out of the blue, not knowing her father and I had been friends for years, was one of life's lovely coincidences.

Before leaving the United States, Smriti had asked if I could bring her a dehydrator, as she was really interested in making more raw foods. We brought her an Excalibur, and Krishna set out to find the right electrical connection.

Madhu and Smriti took us out for a day of shopping, visiting a mosque and the organic market. Mike, Lisa, and I piled in the car, and the driver took off through the packed streets of Delhi. He swerved around cars and people like a skilled surgeon, barely skimming between trucks, buses, small cars, horse-drawn wooden carts, and endless motorcycles. I couldn't look out the front of the car without gasping at every turn, so I turned my head and looked out the side window. Delhi makes New York streets look like deserted roads.

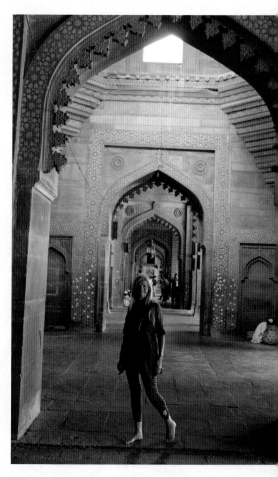

The sites along the way were almost too much to take in: small trucks piled with colorful mattresses, men carrying large filled sacks, women carrying baskets or plastic tubs on their heads, school children in their uniforms coming from class, cardboard houses alongside the road, and women in their beautiful colorful saris brightening up the streets. There was some sort of transformation going on moment to moment, and way too much for the mind to focus on just one thing.

We arrived at Madhu's gallery to admire her truly amazing paintings, which were touched with gold leaf in just the right places. We swooned over paintings of Krishna and his gopi, Goddess Kali, and women in their saris preparing for ceremonies. Madhu had completely captured the spirit, beauty, love, and romance of Lord Krishna in all her paintings.

Across the street, we visited some shops on the way to a mosque. Antiques, fabric, saris, Bollywood posters, and jewelry made us blatantly aware we were in an exotic country.

The mosque was set in a beautiful park, and young lovers appeared to be drawn to this romantic place, with the river below and the peaceful atmosphere. We took lots of photos and left for our next adventure.

Although we have many Indian products imported to stores in America, shopping in India is much more exciting, seeing women buying colorful cord to be wrapped into their hair and henna artists applying designs to women's hands, which is a ceremonial art form called mehndi, traditionally used in weddings. I turned down both, although I did experience mehndi at Rakesh and Deepti's wedding.

We looked at rugs, scarves, shoes, saris and some cotton leggings, which I purchased along with a few gifts for my family. We stopped to sample a piece of yam that was made over hot covered coals. The vendor cut off bite-size pieces, squeezed lime and spices on top, and added pieces of a small, tart star fruit to the paper tray.

We watched several women in saris dance on an outside stage. They had sticks in each hand and were doing a tribal dance called kolattam or "the stick dance." Women danced in a circle and received strikes on their sticks while doing simple steps. The music was typical Indian, and the sticks added to the beat. The performance was reminiscent of a game we played as girls, in which we chanted a rhyme while clapping our own hands together, then slapped our thighs, and then met our partner's hands. The rhyme went faster and faster, and so did the clapping. Somehow the Indian dance felt familiar.

I was convinced to try another nonraw snack at a small stand. It's not something I would do on my own, but with my friends pointing out which stands are okay to eat at, I felt safe, especially knowing there was no raw food for me anywhere in sight. We tried a small veggie dumpling with the hottest sauce I've ever tasted. My eyes teared up, and I quickly grabbed my water bottle. The next was a small puffy ball made with a grain and obviously fried, and when pierced with a fork, it exposed its hollow center. Smirti filled the center with chopped vegetables and lime water. This tidbit had to be put whole in one's mouth all at once so the lime juice does not leak out. I realized I was eating food that has been off my diet for many years, but rather than fret, I looked at it as an experiment and a way to figure out raw Indian food recipes.

After hours of shopping, night fell, and we visited a large marketplace selling everything imaginable. We went there especially for the organic market. The arrangement of stalls was beautiful. The green section was filled with the darkest variety of fresh greens, some of which were familiar, and others I needed to ask about. The fruits were ripe, fresh, and very colorful. Mike was constantly clicking his camera to capture all he could of our experience and the array of fresh produce.

We met up with the rest of the family at a Southern Indian restaurant. Krishna, his son Kunal and daughter Prarthna, Rakesh, and Deepti joined us. After looking over the menu, I saw I was in for another nonraw meal. I already tried cooked food earlier that day, so I decided to see what was in store for me. I had always managed to find something raw in all my travels, but this time I found it much more difficult. Salads were not a good option to eat as they were washed in local water.

I decided on a flat pancake with vegetables. All kinds of hot sauces arrived at the table, and nothing on anyone's plate looked familiar. My cooked dish didn't look too harmful; at least it was vegan. It was delicious and gave me an idea for one of my raw Indian recipes.

As good as it tasted, the dish was not worth the feeling I had the next morning. I hadn't had arthritic pains since I started eating raw foods, but that morning they were back. My knees and hands were stiff and ached. I even had a headache. I think it was good for me to experience again why I continue to eat a raw food diet.

The next day we visited Old Delhi with Madhu and Smirti. Madhu's driver left us at the entrance to Old Delhi. The main street, know as Chandni Chowk, is one of the oldest bazaars in Delhi, with vendors of various merchandise selling their wares. Old Delhi is densely populated and is the heart of Islamic metropolitan Delhi. It is a must-see. Many tourists go through Old Delhi by rickshaw only. But to experience the real feeling, we walked through the maddeningly crowded streets. Electrical wires hung overhead in a maze on every street like tangled-up spaghetti. The streets were uneven, and at each corner's crossing, we had to watch our step. The sidewalk (so to speak) was very narrow with wall-to-wall people. Vendors were in tiny shops, some lined with cushions so customers could go in and sit while they were shown saris, jewelry, or clothes and other goods.

It felt like chaos beyond belief, but it is everyday real life for most people living in Delhi. It was a feast for the body, mind, and spirit. The sounds, smells, and sights flashed by as we rushed towards the spice streets where Madhu bought her spices, nuts, and flours. I knew we were close to the spices because my throat began to tickle and I began to cough. I realized I was not the only one coughing and sneezing. All around me I heard others with the same reaction. The smell was not subtle.

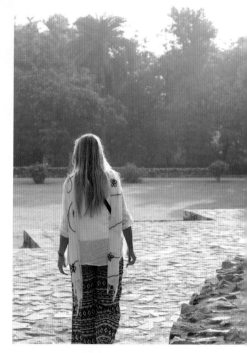

After Madhu bought her spices, she suggested that we take a rickshaw bicycle to leave the area. I felt we were in for another experience I'd never forget. Lisa, Smriti, and I hopped into one bicycle rickshaw, and Mike and Madhu in another. I was hanging on to anything I could get a hold of, as it was a wild bumpy ride. I looked behind but didn't see Mike and Madhu's rickshaw any longer. When they finally showed up, we found out that their rickshaw got caught up with another bicycle rickshaw and a wooden cart carrying a pile of goods. The drivers all had to dismount to shake, twist, and turn their vehicles to untangle the mess. The look on Mike's face was priceless.

We explored New Delhi a couple more days, and then Smirti and Kunal escorted us on the grand tour of Jaipur and Agra. The ride to Jaipur was a complete assault on the senses. While our driver navigated the crowded roads towards our destination, we heard the constant sound of horns honking and watched men and women piled into trucks, four to five members of a family on one motorcycle, and cars driving in the wrong direction on the wrong side of the road. It was beautiful, mesmerizing, and scary all at once.

I would not hesitate to say that of all our travels, nothing could compare with the experience of India. Along the way to Jaipur, we visited a temple, which we were told housed one of the largest Ganesha statues in India. In Jaipur we toured forts and saw elephants, snake charmers, camels, monkeys, sacred cows, and oxen roaming the streets everywhere. Of course, we also shopped. Jaipur, the largest city in Rajasthan, is known for carpets, fabrics, handicrafts, and jewelry. Lisa was having the time of her life shopping for Indian shoes, garments, and a few gifts. Jaipur is a beautiful city with pink-colored stucco-like buildings and walls. I got the feeling it must have been very grand in the early days. Although much modernization had arrived in Jaipur, the old section still stole my heart.

Smriti took Lisa and me to her longtime family astrologer in Jaipur. We were escorted to a tiny room to wait. Soon a small, sweet-looking older man entered the room with his son, who was following in his father's footsteps. Lisa went first and was amazed at his accuracy about her past. She, of course, was interested in her future, which he proceeded to tell her. She received some instructions and a small packet to put under her pillow. Next was my turn, and Smriti translated for me as she had done for Lisa. I was told several things about my past, and everything was accurate. The astrologer said I should surround myself with green. I immediately thought of all my green drinks and garden. He also told me I would live to be at least 100. Since he had been accurate about my past, I took what he said to heart. He saw my life as a very happy one and gave me some instructions to follow. We left feeling very satisfied.

Of course, no trip to Northern India could be complete without visiting Agra to see the Taj Mahal, a breathtaking sight of a white marble mausoleum built by Mughal emperor Shah Jahan in memory of his third wife, who died during the birth of their fourteenth child. We saw the magnificent view of the Taj through the great arched gate. The closer we got, the more beautiful the Taj looked with its intricate white inlaid marble panels. We were all struck with its beauty both inside and out.

After a few days' visit to Agra, we returned back to Delhi to spend the balance of our trip with the rest of the Guptas, do some last minute gift shopping, and reminisce about our past. Mike, Lisa, and I agreed that without our friends taking care of us throughout our trip to India, we would never have experienced this amazing country in the same way. India is one fascinating country!

spices of india

India is a culturally diverse country, and cuisines vary from region to region. Rich scents wafted up from burlap bags on the spice street of Old Delhi. My friend bought her spices from different vendors. She knew which spices were best to buy from each stall. India produces many spices locally. Although some spices were originally imported from other places with similar climates, India has been cultivating these for centuries locally.

My friends taught me years ago that the trick to Indian food is the spices and how they are treated in cooking to bring out their flavors. They are heated in a pan with a drop of ghee or oil to open up the flavors before the food is added. Curry is a combination of several spices blended together. Indian spices and herbs include ginger, cardamom, star anise, cinnamon, turmeric, garam masala, coriander, chili, nutmeg, tamarind, asafetida (or hing), cumin, fenugreek leaf, saffron, garlic, and cloves.

Indians claim certain spices are helpful in dealing with cancer and other diseases. Examples include turmeric, curcumin, fennel, saffron, cumin, cinnamon, cayenne pepper, ginger, anise, garlic, caraway, mint, and oregano.

I've tried to incorporate many of these herbs in my recipes, but feel free to add any extras you feel, especially if you like spicier versions.

Āp Kā Khānā Sv Ādista ho (Enjoy Your Meal)

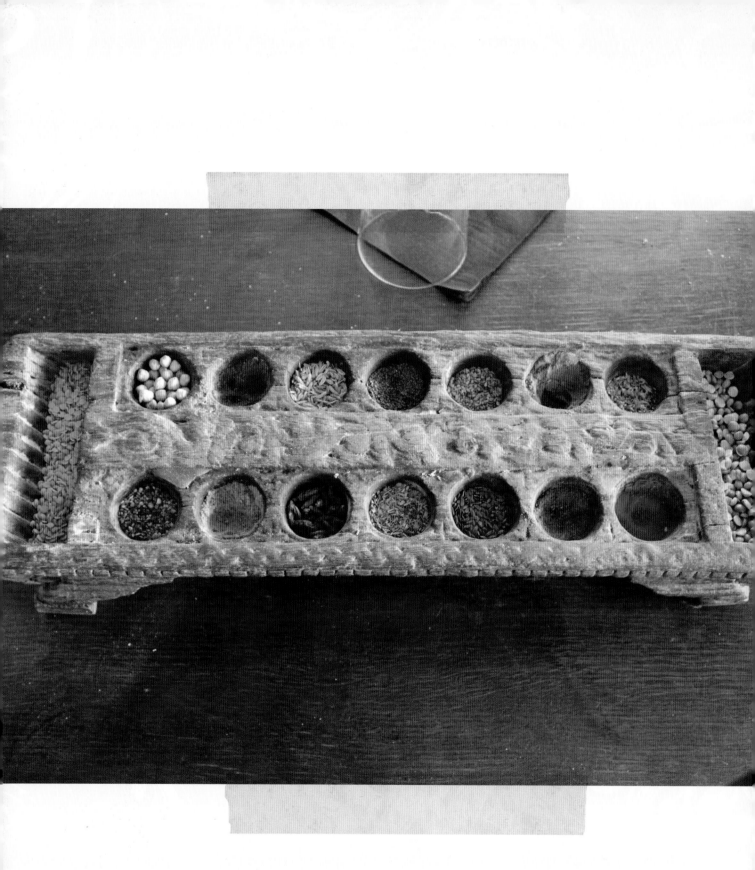

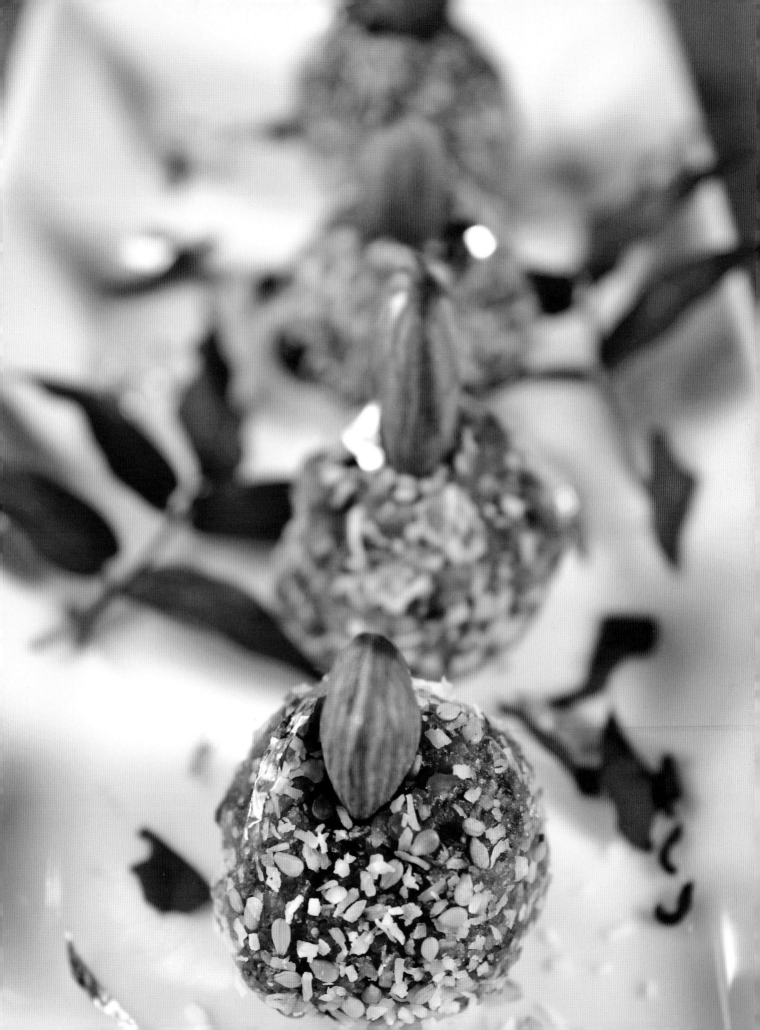

Breakfast (Nashta)

A variety of foods are served for breakfast depending what region you are from. Idli, vadai, dosa, upama, stuffed parathas, and pongal are all popular breakfast dishes, served with chutneys, dhal, and curries. All these dishes are made with flours I just couldn't match. However, any of the dishes in this Indian section are acceptable for breakfast. Biryani with mango curry sauce or coconut yogurt will get your day started with a bang. Halwa is another good breakfast dish (see the desserts section below).

Thinly sliced or chunky-cut mangos, papaya, or bananas are popular fruits for breakfast and what I consumed most mornings along with Rakesh's green drink.

Rakesh's Morning Green Drink

Neem leaves are very bitter but have many medicinal properties. They are more than likely not available in most stores except possibly in Indian markets. I will substitute kale in this drink for the neem leaves, but you won't get the full bitter effect.

1 cup kale leaves (if you find neem leaves, use only a couple)

1 large tomato

1 cucumber

1 inch ginger

1 clove garlic

½ cup gooseberries (if not available, use cranberries)

Water as needed

DIRECTIONS

Juice or blend the ingredients in a high-powered blender, adding water until the mixture becomes smooth. If your blender does not make smooth drinks, strain through a nut filter bag or cheesecloth.

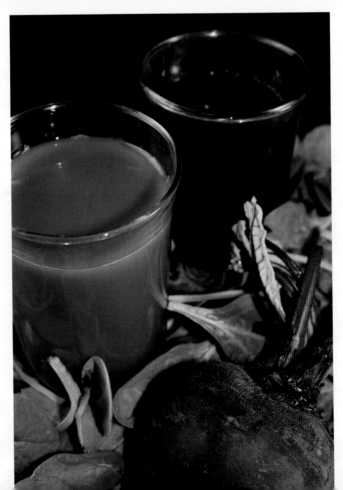

Deepti's Morning Drink

Bottle gourd is another item hard to find in American markets. I am going to use a summer squash, zucchini.

1 cup beet root	½ cup gooseberries or cranberries
1 cup carrots	1 inch ginger
1 cup spinach	1 clove garlic
½ cup zucchini	Water as needed

DIRECTIONS

Juice or blend the ingredients in a high-powered blender, adding water until the mixture becomes smooth. If your blender does not make smooth drinks, strain through a nut filter bag or cheesecloth.

Masala Chai

(2 servings)

2 cardamom pods, crushed	1 cinnamon stick, broken in half
⅛ teaspoon black pepper	1 cup almond milk (see p. 65)
3 whole cloves	2 tablespoons sweetener of choice
½ teaspoon fresh ginger, or ⅛ teaspoon powdered	1½ teaspoons black tea leaves
	1 cup water

DIRECTIONS

Place all ingredients in a mason jar except the milk and tea leaves, and place the jar on the bottom shelf of a dehydrator. Dehydrate at 110° F for approximately 4 hours or until warm. After the mixture is warm, add the milk and tea leaves, place the jar back in the dehydrator, and let warm thoroughly. Strain through a sieve, and discard the spices. The mixture can also be heated in a pan on the stove, but be sure not to overheat. Check constantly with a teaspoon to make sure the temperature does not get too high. The mixture can also be made the evening before, refrigerated overnight, and warmed in the morning. This gives the spices time to permeate the milk and water.

Lunch (Ratri)

Papadum crackers with curry cheese is a great dish to serve along with a salad for lunch or use as an appetizer or snack.

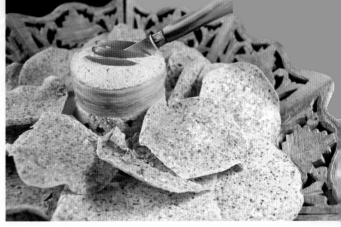

Papadum Crackers with Curry Cheese

(approx. 20 crackers)

2 cups corn kernels	½ teaspoon cumin, ground
¼ cup onion	1 garlic clove, crushed
¼ cup tomato	Himalayan salt to taste
¼ cup flax meal	Water as needed
½ cup sunflower seeds, ground to meal	Chili powder to taste (optional)
½ teaspoon black pepper, freshly milled	

DIRECTIONS

In a high-speed blender, blend the corn, onion, tomato, and ½ cup water. Blend until smooth. Scrape the mixture into a bowl. Sift the flax meal and sunflower meal into bowl, and add the remaining ingredients. Add water as needed to make a wet fluid mixture. Taste for seasonings, and add more if needed. Place the mixture on a nonstick dehydrator sheet one teaspoonful at a time. Leave room between each cracker as the crackers will spread. When the tray is complete, tap one side of it on the kitchen counter, turning to tap each flat side until the crackers are thinned out. Size is your choice. Dehydrate at 115° F for 2–3 hours, then turn over onto a mesh sheet, and carefully lift off the nonstick sheet. If the center sticks, use a knife to help loosen. Dehydrate for another 6 or more hours until the crackers snap and are crispy.

CURRY CHEESE

1 cup sunflower seeds, soaked for 4 hours	1 teaspoon cumin
1 cup pumpkin seeds, soaked for 4 hours	¼ teaspoon coriander
1 tablespoon shallots, chopped	¼ teaspoon turmeric
½ cup red sweet pepper, chopped	Himalayan salt to taste
¼ cup carrots, chopped	1 tablespoon olive oil
1 clove garlic, crushed	½ tablespoon maple syrup or sweetener of choice
1 teaspoon ginger, grated	Chili powder to taste (optional)
Curry powder to taste (1 or more teaspoons)	Water as needed

DIRECTIONS

Drain and rinse the sunflower and pumpkin seeds. Grind them in a blender, adding as little water as necessary to make a smooth thick paste. Place the rest of the ingredients in a food processor and pulse chop, stopping to scrape the sides down as needed. Add the seeds, and chop all ingredients well. Place a strainer over a bowl, and line it with cheesecloth. Place the cheese mixture in the cloth, and fold the cheesecloth over the top. Place a weight or bowl of water on top to help push out any liquid. Leave for several hours. Refrigerate the cheese so it firms up. Serve with papadum crackers and tamarind sauce (see p. 189).

Green Bean Curry

(2–3 servings)

3 cups string beans, cut into 2-inch pieces

1 tablespoon olive oil

½ cup onion, chopped

1 large tomato, chopped

1 clove garlic, crushed

1 teaspoon ginger, grated

½ teaspoon mustard seeds

1 teaspoon cumin seeds, crushed

½ teaspoon turmeric

Chili powder to taste

½ teaspoon curry powder

2 tablespoons fine unsweetened coconut flakes

Himalayan salt to taste

Freshly milled pepper to taste

DIRECTIONS

Place all ingredients except the string beans into a shallow baking dish. Stir to combine. Add the string beans, and mix well to coat. Add more oil if necessary. Spread the string beans out on a nonstick dehydrator sheet, and dehydrate at 115° F for 2–3 hours or until the strings slightly soften. This dish is delicious served with a side dish of biryani (see p. 187). Chutney may also be served.

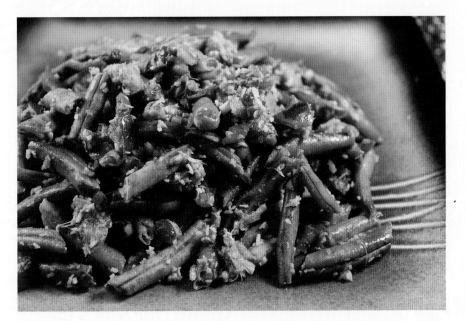

Vegetable Cutlets with Curry Dipping Sauce

(2–3 servings)

1 cup corn kernels

½ cup carrot, pulp or grated

½ cup spinach, chopped

½ cup cabbage, grated

¼ cup onion, chopped

½ teaspoon turmeric powder

Green chili to taste (optional)

¼ teaspoon curry powder

1 cup sunflower seeds

1 cup pumpkin seeds, ground to flour

Water as needed

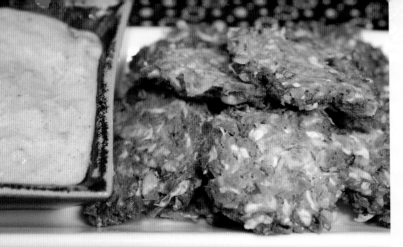

Place the corn and onion in a food processor, and pulse chop until blended. Add the remaining ingredients to a mixing bowl, and blend together. Add water if necessary to make a thick mixture that will hold together. Take a scoop of the mixture and make a ball, then flatten it into a cutlet, about 3 inches in diameter and ½ inch thick. Place all cutlets on a nonstick dehydrator sheet, and dehydrate at 110° F for 2 hours. Turn onto a mesh screen, and remove the nonstick sheet. Continue dehydrating for another 2 hours.

CURRY SAUCE

(approx. 1 cup)

½ cup cashews, soaked for 4 hours	1 teaspoon cumin, ground
1 tablespoon olive oil	⅛ teaspoon turmeric, ground
½ cup onion, chopped	⅛ teaspoon cinnamon powder
1 large tomato, seeded and chopped	⅛ teaspoon black pepper, freshly milled
½ cup fresh cilantro leaves	Himalayan salt to taste
½ teaspoon ginger, grated	Serrano chili to taste, minced (optional)
1 garlic clove, crushed	¼ cup coconut yogurt
1 teaspoon coriander, ground	Water as needed

DIRECTIONS

Place the oil in a bowl, and add the onion, tomato, cilantro, ginger, garlic, coriander, cumin, turmeric, cinnamon, salt, and pepper. Toss until all ingredients are coated.

Spread the mixture on a nonstick dehydrator sheet, and dehydrate at 110° F for 1 hour or until softened. Place the ginger, garlic, and remaining spices in a food processor. Add the softened onion and tomato mixture, and pulse chop until well combined. Add the yogurt and pulse again. Add water as needed to make a medium-thick sauce, and pulse chop a couple of times. Taste for seasonings, and adjust if necessary.

TIP This sauce can be used for rice or as a raw vegetable dip.

MANGO CURRY SAUCE

1 medium mango	1 teaspoon garam masala
¾ cup cashews, soaked	2–3 tablespoons gluten-free tamari
1½ teaspoons curry powder	¾ cup water
½ teaspoon turmeric	½ cup olive oil

DIRECTIONS

Place the cashews and water in a high-powered blender, and blend until smooth, adding more water if needed. Add the remaining ingredients, and blend well. The mixture may be warmed in dehydrator at 110° F for 1 hour and served in combination with the other Indian dishes in this section.

Dinner (Bhojan)

Dinner and lunch recipes are often interchangeable.

Vegetable Biryani

I like this dish for lunch or dinner. It also works well with curry dishes. My friend Rakesh made us an amazing vegetable biryani one evening. When all the spices were brought to their peak and all the vegetables were chopped, he placed everything in the pot, poured the uncooked rice in, and put the lid on. He then sealed the pot with a dough-like substance to keep all the steam in. The dish was really delicious, but it wasn't raw, so I had to figure out a substitute.

MY RAW BIRYANI VERSION

(2–3 servings)

2 cups sprouted wild rice (see p. 44) or parsnip rice (p. 200)

1 cup carrots, finely chopped

1 cup string beans, finely chopped

1 cup sweet peas

1 cup tomatoes, seeded and chopped

1 cup onions, thinly sliced

½ teaspoon mustard seeds

¼ teaspoon fennel seeds

½ teaspoon fenugreek seeds

Pinch of clove powder

⅛ teaspoon cinnamon

4 cardamom seeds, ground

¼ teaspoon coriander powder

¼ teaspoon turmeric powder

½ garam masala

½ teaspoon cumin

3 threads saffron, soaked in 1 tablespoon warm water

½ cup almonds or cashews, chopped

⅛ teaspoon clove powder

½ cups raisins, soaked until soft

Jalapeño pepper, seeded, sliced, to taste (optional)

Himalayan salt to taste

2 tablespoons olive oil

DIRECTIONS

If using wild rice, sprout it the evening before preparing the recipe. Place the carrots, string beans, peas, tomatoes, and onions in a bowl, and toss with 1 tablespoon olive oil. Add all spices, and toss to coat the vegetables. Spread on a nonstick dehydrator sheet, and dehydrate at 110° F for 1½ hour or until soft. While the vegetables are softening, place the rice in a dish, cover with foil, and heat in a dehydrator. When the vegetables are finished, toss with the rice. If you have coconut yogurt on hand (see p. 160), make some raita and serve it with the biryani.

Raita

1 cup coconut yogurt (see p. 160)

1 cup English cucumber, peeled, seeded, and finely chopped

½ teaspoon cumin

Tiny pinch of garlic powder

Himalayan salt to taste

DIRECTIONS

Mix all ingredients in a large bowl, and refrigerate to chill.

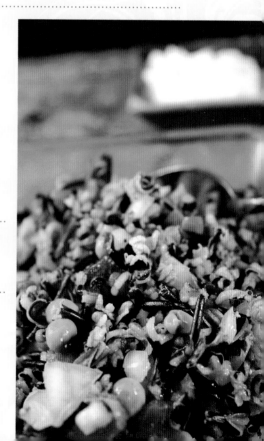

Adraki Gobi, Raw Style

(1–2 servings)

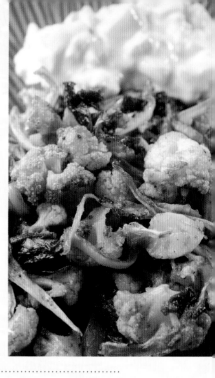

1 cup onion, thinly sliced

1 cup tomato, chopped

2 cups cauliflower, small florets only

1 teaspoon turmeric

Himalayan salt to taste

1 teaspoon ginger, grated

2 teaspoons garam masala

2 tablespoons olive oil

DIRECTIONS

Place the vegetables and spices in a bowl. Toss with olive oil. Place on a nonstick dehydrator sheet, and dehydrate at 110° F for 2–3 hours. Serve with raita.

Pakoras

(approx. 20 balls)

½ cup parsnip, roughly chopped

½ cup sweet potato

½ cup onion, roughly chopped

½ cup carrots, roughly chopped

½ cup bok choy or spinach, roughly chopped

½ cup red bell pepper, roughly chopped

Water if needed

1 tablespoon olive oil

½ teaspoon cumin

½ teaspoon turmeric

½ teaspoon coriander

1 teaspoon garam masala

½ teaspoon curry powder

Chili powder to taste, or jalapeño, chopped (optional)

Freshly milled pepper to taste

Himalayan salt to taste

½ teaspoon ginger, grated

1 clove garlic, crushed

½ cup flax meal (¼ cup flaxseeds makes ½ cup meal)

½ cup sesame seeds, ground to meal (¼ cup sesame seeds makes ½ cup meal)

½ cup sunflower seeds, ground to meal (¼ cup sunflower seeds makes ½ cup meal)

¼ cup almond flour (see p. 45)

DIRECTIONS

Place all vegetables in a food processor, and chop them into small pieces. Transfer the pieces in a mixing bowl. Add the olive oil and spices, and combine well. Add all seed flours, and blend well. If the mixture doesn't hold together when squeezed, add a little water at a time to hold the mixture together when rolled into a ball. Shape the entire mixture into balls, and place the balls directly on a mesh dehydrator sheet. Dehydrate at 110° F for 5–6 hours or longer if preferred. A crust will form on the outside, and the center will be slightly soft.

TO SERVE

Serve with tamarind sauce (see recipe following).

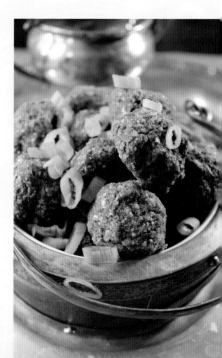

TAMARIND SAUCE

Tamarind may be purchased in Asian markets or some health food stores. It will be either dried or fresh.

- 2–3 tablespoons tamarind pulp
- ½ cup coconut sugar or sweetener of choice
- ¼ cup raisins
- 1 teaspoon cumin
- ½ teaspoon ginger, grated, or ginger powder
- 1 teaspoon garam masala
- Salt and pepper to taste
- Chili powder or pepper flakes to taste (optional)
- 1 cup warm water

DIRECTIONS

Soak the tamarind in warm water for about 15–20 minutes. Mash the pulp, then place a strainer over a bowl and pour the tamarind mixture in. Continue mashing and pressing the pulp into the bowl. Discard any fibers or seeds left in the strainer. Add the remaining ingredients, and mix well. Taste for seasonings and sweetness, and adjust if necessary.

Dessert (Mishti)

CARROT HALWA

Different from the Mediterranean dessert called halva, this dish is more like a thick pudding. There are many different ways to make this dish depending on the region from which a recipe originates. This dish can be served warm or cold. It also makes a great breakfast dish.

- 2 cups carrots, grated
- 2 cups almond milk (see p. 65)
- ½ cup coconut sugar or sweetener of choice
- 1 tablespoon coconut oil
- ¼ cup raisins, soaked
- ¼ cup almonds or cashews, chopped
- 2 cardamom pods, ground to powder, or ¼ cardamom, ground
- 2 tablespoons chia seeds, ground to meal

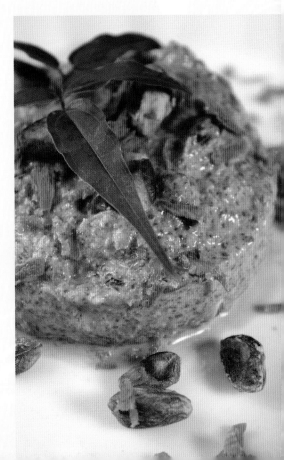

DIRECTIONS

Add the milk and carrots to a food processor, and pulse chop to blend. Add the sweetener, coconut oil, and pulse chop to incorporate. Remove the mixture to a bowl, and add the nuts and raisins. Stir in the ground chia powder. Stir with a whisk to mix the chia, let sit for 10 minutes, and then stir again, breaking up any lump.

TO SERVE

The dish may be warmed in a dehydrator to enjoy on a cold day or served chilled.

Sweet Sesame Seed Balls

2 cups almonds

½ cup sesame seeds

2 cups water

1 teaspoon cardamom powder or seeds ground to powder

5–6 Medjool dates

1 handful pistachio nuts or other nuts of choice

1 handful of raisins, soaked until soft

½ cup fine coconut, flakes

¼ cup sesame seeds

DIRECTIONS

Place the almonds in a food processor, and pulse chop them into small pieces. Add the dates, and pulse chop until all is well blended. Place the mixture in a mixing bowl. Put the sesame seeds and water in a blender, and blend only a short time as you are going to use the sesame seed pulp. Strain the mixture through a nut milk bag or cheesecloth, and squeeze all water out. Put the sesame pulp in the bowl with almond-date mixture, and mix in well. Add the cardamom and sweetener, and mix again. Crush the pistachio nuts, and mix them in. Drain the raisins, and add them to the mixture. Blend all ingredients well. Taste for seasonings, and add more sweetener if desired. To make small balls, place a bit of mixture in the palms of your hands and roll firmly to create a ball. Mix the shredded coconut and the sesame seeds together on a flat plate. Roll the balls in coconut and sesame seeds to cover. The desert is now ready to eat.

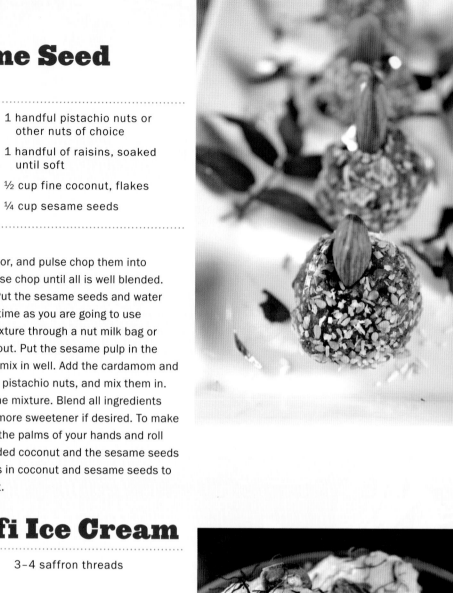

Saffron Kuifi Ice Cream

½ cup pistachios

2 cups almond milk (see p. 65)

3–4 saffron threads

DIRECTIONS

In a small bowl, soak the saffron threads in 1 tablespoon of warm water for 5 minutes. Chop the pistachios roughly, and reserve a few to chop finely for garnish. Mix the nuts into the almond milk, and add the saffron with water. Pour the mixture in a jar, and refrigerate it for 4–5 hours. If you have an ice cream maker, pour in the mixture and follow the manufacturer's directions. Remove the ice cream by the tablespoon or ice cream scoop, and shape it onto parchment paper that is placed in a baking dish. Place the ice cream in a freezer until firm and ready to serve. If you don't have an ice cream maker, freeze the mixture until it is just firm enough to remove with a tablespoon or ice cream scoop, and shape it onto parchment paper. When the ice cream is firm, serve it with chopped nuts on top. Store it in a closed container in a freezer.

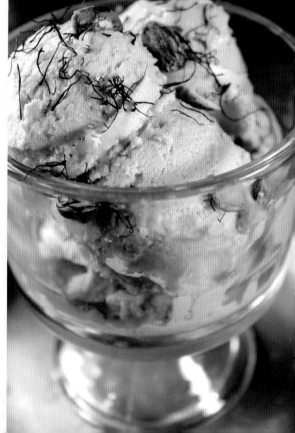

Mango Lassi

1 large mango

¼–½ teaspoon cardamom powder

Pinch of cinnamon

1 cup coconut yogurt (see p. 160), or ¾ cup almond milk and ½ avocado

½ cup ice cubes

Sweetener to taste

DIRECTIONS

Place all ingredients in a high-speed blender, and blend until smooth. Pour the mixture in a milk bag, and strain. Serve in chilled glasses.

Orange Milk

6 ounces fresh orange juice

¾ cup almond milk

Sweetener of choice to taste

½ cup water

1 teaspoon vanilla

½ cup ice cubes

DIRECTIONS

Put all ingredients except the ice in a high-speed blender, and blend until smooth. Add the ice, one cube at a time, until desired texture is achieved.

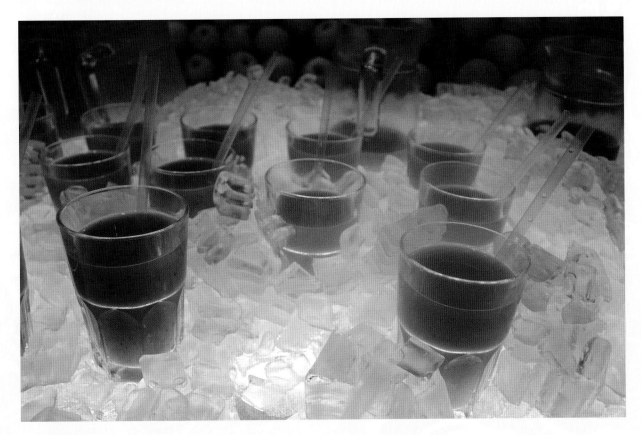

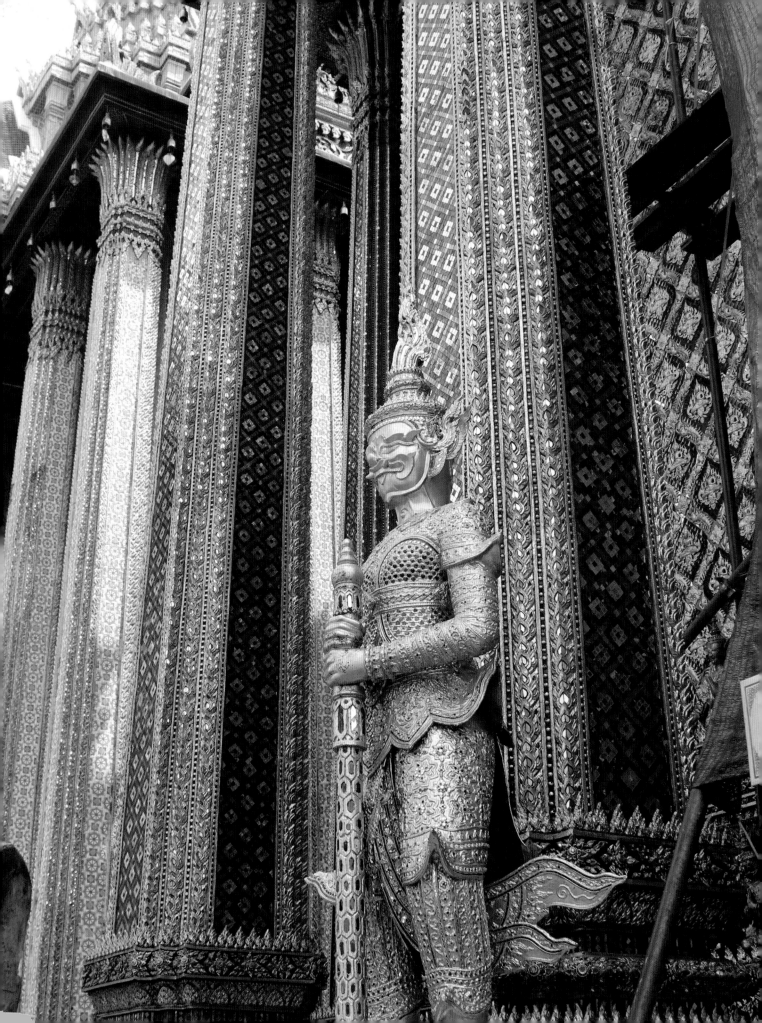

CHAPTER 17

·····················

RAW CUISINE—TASTE OF

THAILAND

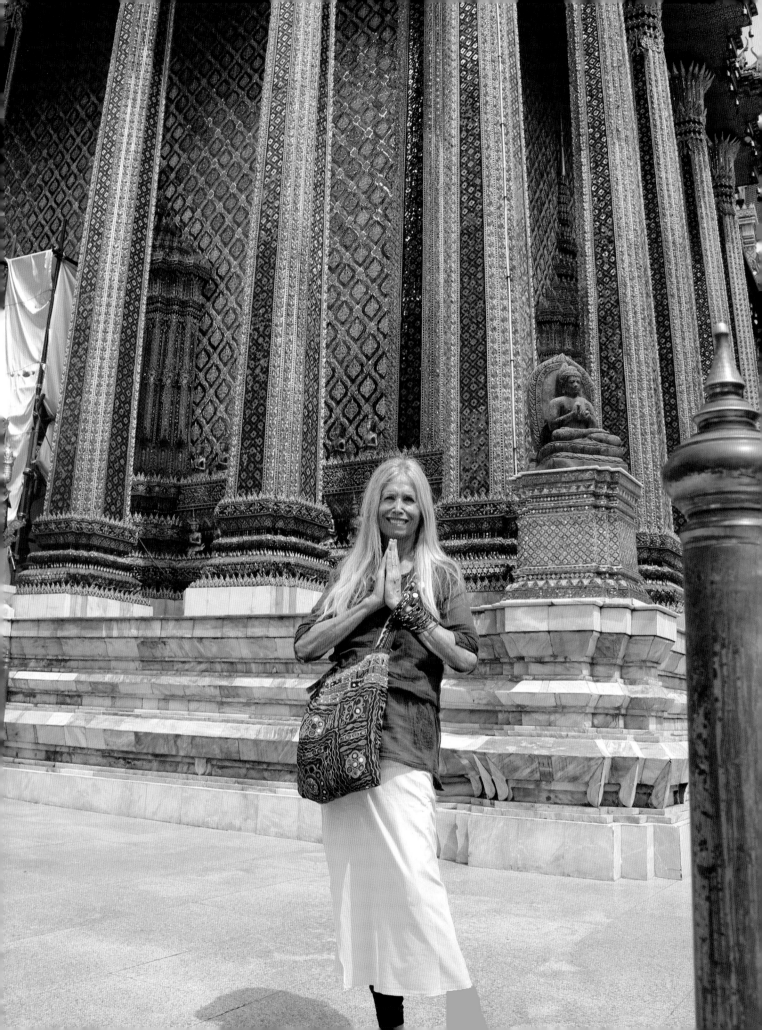

had heard so many great things about Thailand that I couldn't wait to finally experience it firsthand. Deciding which city was not easy, but since Bangkok is the capital of Thailand and we have friends who live there, we decided this would be the place to visit.

Many raw foodists love Thailand because fruits are bountiful. Thai fruits are exported to specialty stores around the world but are commonly found in every marketplace in Thailand. Prices are low and the quality very high.

I knew Bangkok was a modern city, but I didn't expect to see so many high-rise buildings and world-class hotels. Yet, even though Bangkok is growing rapidly, it manages to preserve its cultural heritage. Bangkok has many historic temples that are beautiful beyond belief. Seeing saffron-robed monks made us feel like time was standing still.

The day after we arrived, our long-time friends Sunny and Yupin picked us up at our hotel to give us an overall view of the city. A sizeable vegetarian festival was going on in Chinatown. Decorations were hanging across the roads, and hundreds of vendors filled the street with vegetarian food stands. I'm always happy to see vegetarianism growing around the world.

We made a stop at the JJ Market (Chatuchak/Jatujak), where one can find the best produce, including all kinds of unusual cooked foods. The smells were larger than life, and on a hot day it was all quite dizzying.

Yupin wanted to make sure we tasted everything locally grown in this agricultural country of tropical fruits. One stand after another, we tasted fresh durian, mangosteen, custard apple, plum mango, gooseberry, guava, jujube, longan, rose apple, rambutan, dragon fruit, lychee, fresh green coconut, regular coconut, and pineapple. All delicious!

We watched women cut fruits into beautiful designs and package them for quick take-away. They looked like pieces of art when they were finished. Everything was ripe, sweet, flavorful, and picked for eating fresh, instead of for shipping. It only took a few bites for me to realize that Thai fruits imported to America do not taste the same as they do in their native land. We tasted brown coconut, green coconut, and my favorite young Thai coconut, which was not frozen as we usually taste it in the United States. One word to describe it: awesome! The cost of a young Thai coconut was about $0.20.

I watched fresh brown coconut being pressed into juice via a three-process method using a machine similar to my new Walker juicer. First, the coconut was fed through a grinding tube. The coconut meat was then placed in a large cloth and moved to a hydraulic press, which extracted the pure liquid into a large container.

After having our fill, we pulled ourselves away from the produce section to cross the street for some shopping. The famous Chatuchak market is a 35-acre home to more than 8,000 market stalls. This market is only open on weekends, and I can't imagine anyone could see the whole market in such a short time. It's truly a shopaholic's delight. Everything and anything you can think of is sold there.

After a good amount of time checking out the stalls and buying a few trinkets, we departed from our dear friends to go back to our hotel and rest. It seemed like a waste of time staying in our room, but a break was necessary as the heat and humidity made us tired. After a short rest, we left for a massage at one of the twenty choices on the street where we were staying. The different kinds of massages offered were vast, and I opted for a foot massage, which is something I could enjoy daily.

The next morning, we headed out to visit the Grand Palace. If there is one place not to miss in Bangkok, this is the place. It was the home of the Thai king and the royal court. The architecture and detail on the many buildings within the walls are dazzling. It is the spiritual heart of Thailand. The Grand Palace has a very strict dress code. I was wearing leggings and a long overshirt but had to rent or purchase a long wraparound skirt. Inside, women are not allowed to bare their shoulders, and men must wear long pants and shirts with sleeves.

We wandered around from building to building awestruck at the fine mosaic work covering every building. We entered a temple and sat on the floor for a time to absorb the gold alter and ornate ceilings. I couldn't recall ever experiencing anything quite like this before. I could feel the energy of all the prayers that have gone on in this temple. We were in a time warp, trying to imagine how buildings like this could have been constructed in 1782.

We spent our final day walking around exploring the local sights and getting ready for my evening talk in front of a group of vegetarians/vegans and raw foodists. In the early evening, we were picked up and taken to the lovely condo building of our hosts, Chef Jennifer M. Robertson and her husband, Kevin. Jennifer, originally from Texas, is a petite woman who was in her ninth month of pregnancy. I learned that Jennifer was trained at Matthew Kenny Academy in Oklahoma and gave raw food classes once a month. You can check her out at "De-hydrated – Modern Living Cuisine" on Facebook.

Jennifer put out many platters of beautifully arranged fruit for our get-together. A very enthusiastic group of men and women began to collect, including a boy of about eleven who was really interested in healthy eating. He proceeded to tell us what kind of smoothies his dad fixed him every day. It was wonderful meeting so many people in Thailand who were on a healthy path. A few brought my book to sign, and others were going to the local international bookstore to purchase it the next morning.

We learned about a retreat called Rasayana, which had a raw food restaurant adjacent to the retreat center. Although we didn't have time to visit, Rasayana seemed like a great place to unwind and clean up one's diet. The center also offers a detox program. I checked out the restaurant menu online, and it offers plenty of great choices for raw dining. On our next trip, we will be sure to visit the place.

Aria Organic Café is another raw food restaurant in Bangkok. It's very small and does not have much seating space, but it has a nice simple menu. There are many vegetarian restaurants in Bangkok, and I can see the interest growing for raw food. Thailand is certainly a place I would like to visit again.

spices

As all in countries, Thai herbs and spices have their own special worldly taste. If you visit a marketplace in this part of the world, you will hardly recognize many of the foods or smells unless it is your place of origin. Spices in Thailand range from sweet to salty to sour. Thai food certainly has a distinct character. Siamese ginger is a very large ginger, much larger and smoother than the ones we find in markets in America, but any Asian market will most likely carry Siamese ginger. Regular ginger is also used, but it's said a good curry paste always uses Siamese ginger. Chilies of many varieties make up chili paste, curry powder, sweet, basil, lemongrass, spring onions, mint, turmeric, lime, kaffir lime leaves, cloves, cumin, nutmeg, garlic, galangal (which is a form of ginger), and shallots (which are preferred over onions). Monosodium glutamate (MSG) is used widely in Thai food, so if you do happen to eat in a Thai restaurant, be sure to ask if the cooks would leave it out of your dish.

Kŏr Hâi Jà-rern Aa-hăan (Enjoy Your Meal)

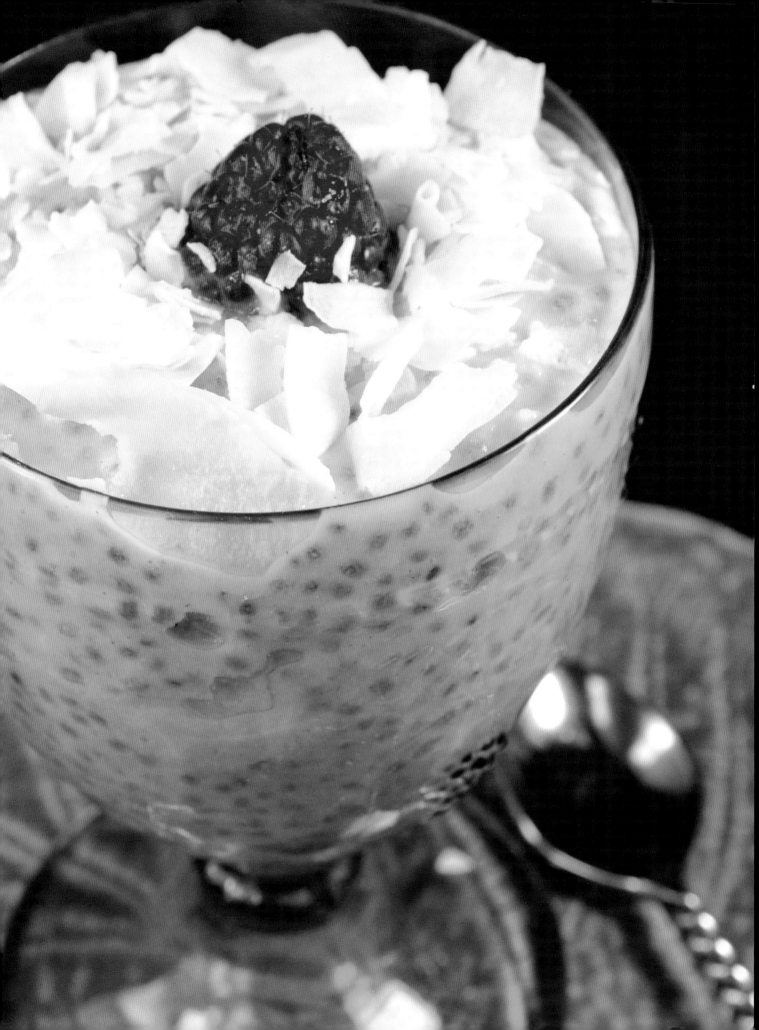

Breakfast (Ahan Chao)

A typical Thai breakfast consists of a thick rice soup with meat called kao tom. It also includes a variety of fried sweets and fruits. I've come up with a breakfast list that I think appropriate for healthy raw vegan dining.

A spicy little morning pick-me-up:

Thai Green Drink with Ginger

1 ripe mango, cut into cubes

2 cups sun green tea

2 packed cups dark leafy greens of choice

2 inches fresh ginger, or to taste, peeled and chopped

½ sweet red bell pepper, roughly chopped

Pinch of cayenne

DIRECTIONS

Place 2 cups water in a jar and add 2 green tea bags. Place in the sun for 4 hours or longer. Remove bags and pour tea into a high-speed blender. Add mango cubes, dark leafy greens, sweet red pepper and blend well. Blend in pinch of cayenne.

TIP Make tea the day before, remove tea bag, and chill in refrigerator or add ice to drink if desired.

Apple, Green Mango, and Seasonal Fruit with Lime

1 cup green apples, seeded and shredded

1 cup green mango, shredded

1 cup fruit in season, thinly sliced (could substitute with mango, pineapple, or coconut flakes)

Juice of 1 lime

1 teaspoon lemon juice

2 tablespoons pomegranate seeds

DIRECTIONS

After shredding the apples, squeeze lemon on top, and mix in to prevent the apples from turning brown. Mix the lime juice in with the green mango and other fruits. Mound on a chilled plate, and garnish with pomegranate seeds.

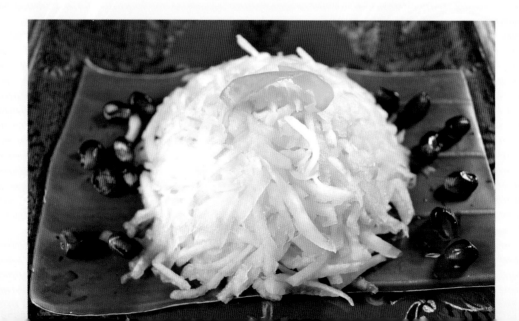

Coconut and Banana Pancakes

(approx. 1 dozen 3-inch pancakes)

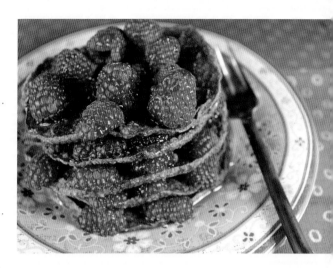

2 ripe bananas

Meat from 1 young Thai coconut

½ cup chia meal, made by grinding chia seeds in spice or coffee grinder

3 tablespoons maple syrup or sweetener of choice

½ cup pecans, finely ground

½ cup oat groats, finely ground

DIRECTIONS

Blend the coconut meat in a food processor or blender, adding enough coconut water to blend smoothly. Add the sweetener, pecans, and ground chia seeds. Blend on low to combine. Add the bananas, groats, and coconut mixture to the food processor, and process until well incorporated. Pour the batter into a bowl. Place a few tablespoons onto a nonstick dehydrator sheet, smoothing into 3-inch pancakes about ½-inch thick. When the entire mixture is used, dehydrate the pancakes at 110° F for 1½ hours, turn the nonstick sheet over onto to a mesh sheet, and carefully peel off the top sheet with the help of a large knife or pastry spatula to separate the sticky part from the sheet. Dehydrate for another 3 hours. The pancakes should have a soft center and a slight crust on the outside.

TO SERVE

Serve the pancakes warm with warm maple syrup and berries.

Pineapple Boat

1 pineapple

Other fruits of choice

Mint leaves

DIRECTIONS

Cut the pineapple in half lengthwise. Cut out the pineapple meat into small pieces. Add 2–3 more fruits that are chopped, or berries of any kind. Chop the mint leaves for a garnish.

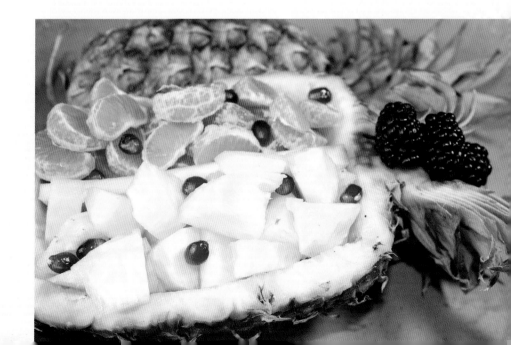

Lunch (Ahan Klang Wan)

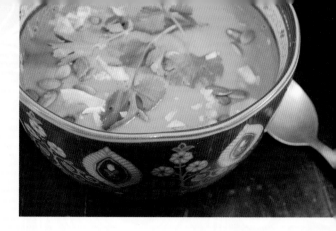

Creamy Pumpkin Coconut Soup

(3–4 servings)

- 1 cup pumpkin, peeled, seeded, and cubed
- 1 cup sweet potato, peeled and cubed
- ½ cup cashews, soaked for 4 hours
- 1 tablespoon to 1 cup water
- Water and meat from young Thai coconut
- 2-inch piece lemongrass, chopped
- 2 kaffir lime leaves
- Pinch of Himalayan salt
- 1 thumbnail-size piece ginger
- 1 tablespoon shallot, chopped
- 4 basil leaves
- 1 spring onion, chopped
- ½ teaspoon cumin
- ½ cup cilantro
- 1 teaspoon lime juice

DIRECTIONS

Blend all ingredients in a high-speed blender, reserving the cashews. Add the drained cashews, blending until mixture is thick and creamy. Top each soup with ribbon-cut basil and ½ teaspoon sesame oil. Warm slightly. Serve the soup in big bowls.

Rice and Pineapple Salad

(2 servings)

Salad

- 2 cups parsnips, peeled
- ½ cup pineapple, chopped
- 2 tablespoons parsley leaves, chopped
- ¼ cup red onion, finely chopped
- ½ cup red bell pepper, finely chopped
- ½ cup raisins or dried cranberries, soaked until soft
- ½ cup whole cashews
- 1 green onion, chopped
- ½ English cucumber, finely chopped, seeds removed
- Pinch of Himalayan salt

DIRECTIONS

In a food processor, chop the parsnip into rice-like pieces. Place in a bowl, add the balance of ingredients, and lightly toss.

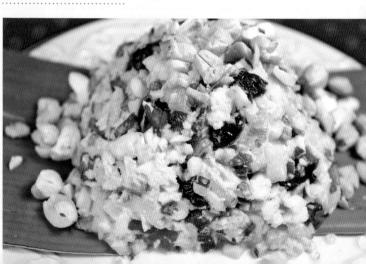

Dressing

½ cup pineapple juice	Small pinch Himalayan salt if needed
1 clove garlic, crushed	1 tablespoon lime juice
1 thumbnail-piece ginger, grated	1 tablespoon maple syrup or sweetener of choice
1 tablespoon sesame oil	
1½ teaspoons tamari or unprocessed miso	4 tablespoons cashews, soaked for 4 hours

DIRECTIONS

Place all ingredients in a blender, reserving the cashews, and blend until smooth. Taste, and adjust the seasonings if necessary. Add the cashews, and blend again until the mixture becomes smooth.

TO ASSEMBLE

Toss the dressing together with the salad, and sprinkle with 1 tablespoon of sesame seeds or whole cashews.

TO SERVE

Serve chilled.

Thai Cucumber Salad

Salad

1 English cucumber, peeled and scored with fork	½ cup basil, chopped
1 red bell pepper, diced	1 cup cilantro, chopped
3 spring onions, thinly sliced	½ cup cashews, chopped

DIRECTIONS

Cut the cucumber in half lengthwise, remove the seeds, and cut into thin slices. Place all salad ingredients in a mixing bowl.

Dressing

1 clove garlic, crushed	⅛–½ teaspoon dried chili flakes
2 tablespoons lime juice	1 teaspoon maple syrup or sweetener of choice
1 tablespoon gluten-free tamari	

DIRECTIONS

Place all dressing ingredients in a bowl, and whisk together. Taste for seasonings, and adjust if necessary.

TO ASSEMBLE

Pour the dressing over the salad, and gently toss. Garnish with black sesame seeds.

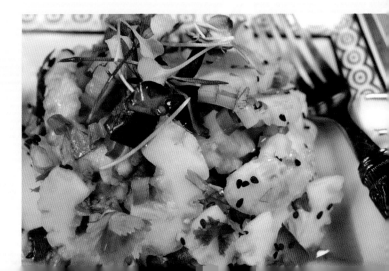

Dinner (Ahan Yen)

Pad Thai Noodles—Salty, Sour, Spicy, and Sweet

(1 serving)

2 cups zucchinis, peeled and spiralized (1 medium zucchini makes about 1 packed cup)

½ cup sweet red pepper, thinly sliced

½ cup per mung bean sprouts

½ cup carrots, thinly sliced with potato peeler

1 spring onion, chopped

¼ cup basil, ribbon cut

¼ cup cilantro leaves

Chopped cashews or sesame seeds, reserved for garnish

DIRECTIONS

Prepare the zucchini; sprinkle a little salt, a squeeze of lemon, and a teaspoon of oil on top. Massage with your fingers, and set the zucchini aside to soften and drain. Prepare the peppers, carrots, and spring onions in the same way.

Sauce

1 cup young Thai coconut meat or 1½ cashews, soaked for 4 hours

1–1½ cup coconut water or purified water

½ cup basil

Juice from one juicy lime

1–2 teaspoons tamari

1–2 cloves garlic, crushed

Small green chili, deseeded and thinly sliced (amount of your choice)

2-inch piece lemongrass, white part only

¼ cup cilantro leaves

½ teaspoon turmeric powder

1 teaspoon ginger, peeled and grated

1 tablespoon almond butter (only if using coconut meat)

1 tablespoon olive oil

Pinch of Himalayan salt

1–2 tablespoons maple syrup or sweetener of choice to taste

Extra basil for garnish

Chopped cashews for garnish

DIRECTIONS

Place all ingredients in a high-speed blender, and blend until smooth, adding water as necessary to make a thick, smooth sauce.

TO ASSEMBLE

Pour the sauce over the vegetables, and mix well. Heat in a dehydrator or in a pan on the stove. Be sure not to overheat. The temperature should be warm and not hot. Chop fresh basil on top, then generously sprinkle whole or chopped cashews.

TO SERVE

Serve with lemon wedges, and chopped cashews on top.

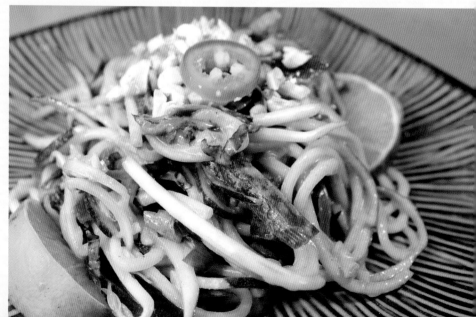

Mung Bean Sprouts with Vegetable Curry
(2 servings)

2 cups mung bean sprouts, rinsed

1–2 cloves garlic, minced

½ cup cabbage, shredded

2 tablespoons sesame oil

4 shiitake mushrooms, thinly sliced

½ cup daikon radish, grated (may substitute with red radish)

1 inch ginger, grated

½ cup bok choy, thinly sliced

1 tablespoon gluten-free tamari

Himalayan salt to taste

2 spring onions, sliced on bias

Sesame seeds for garnish

Mint for garnish

DIRECTIONS

Lightly toss all ingredients together, and spread the mixture on a nonstick dehydrator sheet. Dehydrate for 2 hours at 110° F. Serve warm with a side of rice and tamarind sauce.

Rice

2 cups parsnip

½ cup pine nuts

1 carrot

DIRECTIONS

Pulse chop the parsnips and carrot in a food processor until rice-like pieces are formed. Add the pine nuts, and pulse chop 2–3 times. Place the mixture in a bowl, and toss with 2 teaspoons sesame oil and 1 teaspoon gluten-free tamari. Set aside.

Curry Sauce

1 clove garlic, crushed

1–2 inches ginger, grated

½ teaspoon turmeric

½ teaspoon curry powder

¼ cup basil

¼ cup mint

1 tablespoon gluten-free tamari

1 tablespoon maple syrup or sweetener of choice

½ cup cilantro

1 tablespoon lime juice

1 cup coconut water

1 small jalapeño pepper, seeds removed, or chili flakes to taste

½ avocado for thickener

DIRECTIONS

Blend all ingredients in a high-speed blender until smooth. Taste, and adjust if necessary.

TO ASSEMBLE

Pour the desired amount of warmed curry sauce over the mung bean mixture, and lightly toss. Serve the rice in a small bowl on the side, which may be warmed in a dehydrator.

TO SERVE

Serve the mung bean mixture and sauce warm.

TIP { Curry sauce may also be used for marinated and dehydrated vegetables of your choice.

Wilted Cabbage Spring Rolls

1 head cabbage

2 spring onions, cut lengthwise in thin strips

2 carrots, cut in matchstick pieces

2 cups red cabbage, shredded

½ cup daikon or radish, shredded

¼ cup mint leaves

½ cup basil, ribbon cut

½ English cucumber, seeded and matchstick cut

½ cup cilantro leaves

½ cup cashews, chopped

DIRECTIONS

Purchase a loose cabbage head if possible. Some are packed tightly and are heavier, but a light cabbage usually has looser leaves. Remove the core with a paring knife, and run the leaves under water. Lifting at the core end of the top leaf, carefully remove the leaves one at a time until you have as many leaves as you want to roll. Pat the leaves dry, and pare down on a hard surface as close as you can. Rub the leaves with a tiny drop of olive oil, and set on a nonstick dehydrator sheet. Dehydrate for about 1 hour at 110° F until the cabbage is wilted. In the meantime, prepare the filling and sauces.

Prepare the vegetables, and place them separately on a large plate. In this way you will have control over how much of each vegetable you place on the leaf.

TIP { Boston lettuce leaves or chard leaves also work well, and not dehydrated.

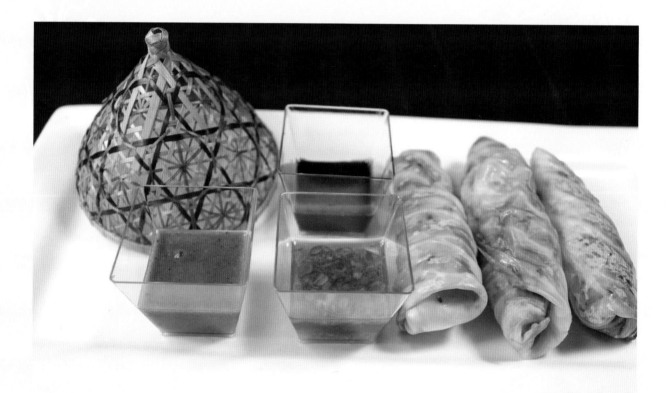

Dipping Sauces

DIPPING SAUCE 1

1 tablespoon apple cider vinegar

4 tablespoons sesame oil

1 tablespoon almond butter

1 tablespoon gluten-free tamari

1 teaspoon maple syrup or
sweetener of choice

DIRECTIONS

Blend all ingredients together with a wire whisk.

DIPPING SAUCE 2

1 tablespoon fresh ginger, grated

1 clove garlic, crushed

1 spring onion, green part only, finely
chopped

1 tablespoon lime juice

Pinch of crushed red pepper flakes,
or to taste

¼ cup water

2 teaspoons apple cider vinegar

1 tablespoon sesame oil

1 teaspoon gluten-free tamari

1 tablespoon maple syrup or
sweetener of choice

DIRECTIONS

Wisk the ingredients together in a bowl, and let the mixture sit for 15 minutes.

TAMARIND SAUCE

*Tamarind can be purchased in Asian markets, most health food stores, or online. Fresh can also be purchased.
I used tamarind paste in a jar.*

½ cup tamarind paste

Pinch of chili flakes, or to taste

1 tablespoon maple syrup or
sweetener of choice

1 tablespoon sesame or olive oil

1 tablespoon gluten-free tamari

1 tablespoon water

DIRECTIONS

Blend all ingredients with a wire whisk. Taste, and adjust to your liking if necessary.

DIRECTIONS FOR WRAP ASSEMBLY

Remove the cabbage leaves from the dehydrator. Lay the softened leaves on a chopping board or plate. Pare down any hard spot that might be left. Place a small amount of each filling on top of each leaf. Drizzle a little tamarind sauce on top of the vegetables. Roll each leaf over once, pull back on the top to secure the filling, then fold the sides in and continue rolling firmly to the end. Place the leaves face down on a plate with the smooth side up. This will help seal the rolls. Continue until all leaves are used. Serve at room temperature with three dipping sauces. Store in a refrigerator.

Desserts

Coconut and Banana Ice Cream

2 cups cashews

1 frozen banana, broken in pieces

2 cups purified water

2 tablespoons coconut oil, melted

1 cup young Thai coconut meat

¼ cup coconut water

½ cup maple syrup or sweetener of choice to taste

½ teaspoon coconut extract or vanilla extract

½ cup medium-size dried coconut flakes, soaked

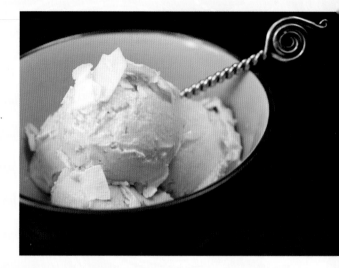

DIRECTIONS

Place all ingredients except the coconut flakes in a high-speed blender, and blend until smooth. Add the coconut flakes, and stir by hand. Pour the mixture into a mason jar or container with a lid, and place it in a refrigerator overnight to meld the flavors. Transfer the mixture to an ice cream maker and follow the manufacturer's directions, or freeze it in a glass baking dish, scraping every ½ hour. The ice cream is ready to eat when frozen but creamy.

Coconut Chia Pudding

1 young Thai coconut, water and meat

1 cup almond or cashew milk (see p. 65)

5 tablespoons chia seeds

2 tablespoons coconut oil, melted

¼ cup unsweetened coconut flakes, medium size

6 tablespoons maple syrup or sweetener of choice

DIRECTIONS

Blend the coconut water and meat in a high-speed blender. Add the coconut oil, and blend again. Place the almond milk and blended coconut mixture in a bowl. Add the chia seeds, and blend with a wire whisk. Let the mixture sit for 10 minutes, and whisk again. Repeat this process 3 more times. Add the sweetener and coconut flakes, and whisk again. Place the mixture in a refrigerator to chill for 5–6 hours or overnight. Garnish with more coconut flakes.

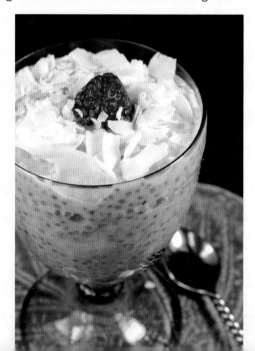

Mango Pudding, Thai Style

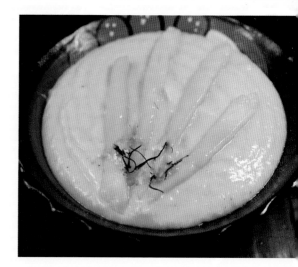

2 mangos

1 tablespoon coconut oil

1 tablespoon maple syrup or sweetener of choice

1 teaspoon lime juice

Meat from 1 young Thai coconut

½ cup young Thai coconut water

½ cup cashews, soaked for 1 hour

Seeds scraped from ½ of a vanilla bean or ½ teaspoon vanilla extract

Generous pinch of cardamom powder

DIRECTIONS

Place all ingredients in a blender, and blend them until smooth. Chill in a refrigerator for 5–6 hours or overnight. Serve in small bowls, and garnish with a saffron thread.

Beverages

Orange and Banana Punch

2 bananas, frozen

2 oranges, peeled and seeded

1 cup ice

2 cups water

4 dates or sweetener of choice

DIRECTIONS

Place all ingredients in a blender, and blend until smooth. Serve in a tall glass, and garnish with an orange slice.

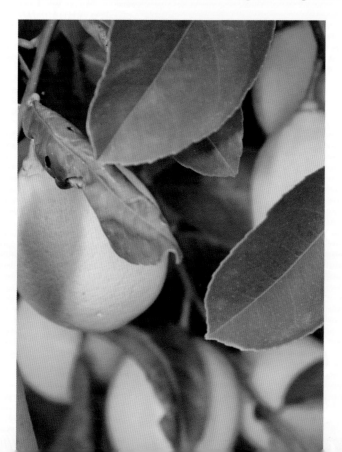

Creamy Thai Tea

1½ cups water

2 teaspoons green tea or 1 tea bag

2 teaspoons maple syrup or sweetener of choice

3 tablespoons cashew milk

½ cup ice

DIRECTIONS

Boil water and let it cool to the touch. Pour it over green tea and let steep 10–15 minutes, or place the tea and water in a jar and leave it in the sun for a few hours. Place all ingredients except the tea bag in a blender, and blend until thick and creamy.

Bubble Tea or Juice

Chia seeds can be added to any juice or tea. Chia seeds are full of protein and give a tapioca-like texture to the drink. It's a very popular Asian drink, classically boiled with tea, tapioca, and sugar.

Ingredients

1–2 tablespoons chia seeds

8 oz glass green tea or juice

½ cup almond milk

Sweetener of choice to taste

DIRECTIONS

Place the seeds in the glass of green tea. Let the seeds swell, stirring several times. Add the milk and sweetener, and stir. Add ice if desired.

FRUIT BUBBLE DRINK

2 tablespoons chia seeds

1 carton organic strawberries, or a 10–12 oz bag frozen organic strawberries, slightly thawed

3 cups water

Sweetener of choice to taste

DIRECTIONS

Place the strawberries, water, and sweetener in a blender, and combine until smooth. Pour into a pitcher, and add chia seeds. Stir with a wire whisk so the seeds do not lump up. Let rest for 5–10 minutes, and stir again. Continue 3–4 more times until seeds are swollen. Add crushed ice, and pour into tall glasses. Add a large-opening straw, and garnish with a strawberry on the rim of each glass.

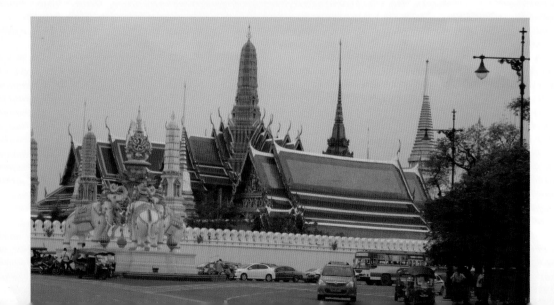

Resources

WHERE TO PURCHASE ORGANIC SPICES, HERBS, AND EXTRACTS

If you don't have a health food store nearby or you can't find an ingredient needed for a recipe, I've included a few online companies I personally use. You can also find the products and equipment I use on my website www.youngonrawfood.com by going to "shop" at the top of the menu bar for the best-tasting and purest organic flavorings, extracts, oils, and many other wonderful products.

MEDICINE FLOWER

For organic spices and herbs:
www.medicineflower.com/flavorextracts.html

SMITH & TRUSLOW

For bulk organic spices and herbs, plus many other products:
www.smithandtruslow.com

STARWEST BOTANICALS

For bulk herbs, spices, extracts, and oils:
www.starwest-botanicals.com/category/bulk-organic-herbs/

SPROUTHOUSE

For organic oat groats and a host of other sprouting products:
www.sprouthouse.com/Oat_Groats_RAW_p/oatgr.htm

SHOP ORGANIC

For all general products:
www.shoporganic.com

THE RAW FOOD WORLD STORE

For all general products:
http://therawfoodworld.com/

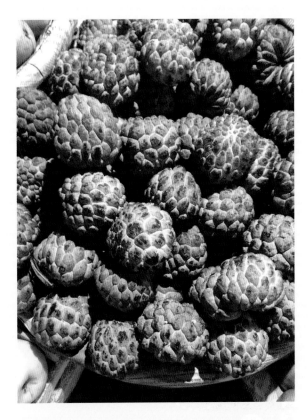

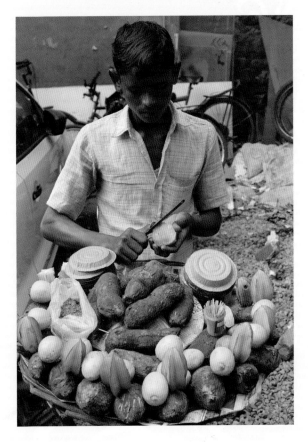

Become a Raw Food Chef

MATTHEW KENNY ACADEMY (SANTA MONICA)

www.matthewkenneycuisine.com

LIVING LIGHT INSTITUTE

http://rawfoodchef.com

INSTITUTE FOR INTEGRATIVE NUTRITION

www.integrativenutrition.com/go/raw/

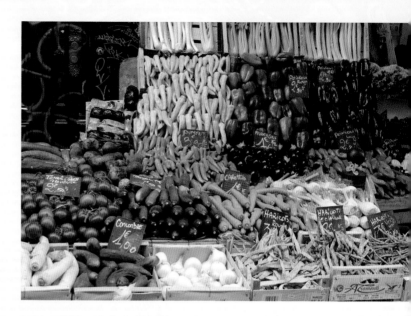

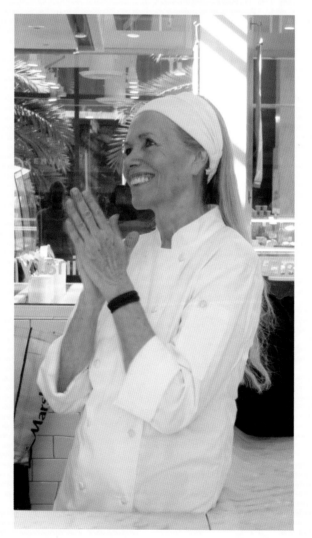

Acknowledgments

There are so many people to thank, so let me start with my partner, Mike Mendell, whom I mention throughout the book. Mike, you are my rock. No words can express my respect and thanks for all you do for me daily. Without your amazing photos to bring all the recipes alive, this would be a very dull-looking book.

Thanks to my family, who have always been my biggest cheerleaders. My children, Dan, Lisa, Jonas, and Mia; my beautiful grandchildren, Mackenzie, Hannah, Karly, Rocky, Luke, Audrey, and Gunner—I love you all so much; and my sisters, Arlene and Sydell, who always let me know they are proud of their sister.

To all my social-network friends on Facebook, Twitter, and LinkedIn: Because of all your support helping to make my first book, *Live Raw*, such a success, *Live Raw Around the World* was made possible. Thank you all for your constant inspiration.

I'm lucky to have the support of good friends who always root for me, including Julie Kavner, my best girlfriend for many years; my dear friend Robin Leach, who is always so generous with his praise of my raw food lifestyle; Susan Santilena, my close friend who is always willing to help me with all my endeavors; Michael Keller and Eileen Chousa Katzenstein, who traveled with us to help gather photos and information for the book; my neighborhood gang, who is always happy to try out my new concoctions; and xoxox to Jim Pross, who graciously helped me edit the manuscript.

I want to thank my agent, Kari Stuart, who has been a great support from day one, when she read my first manuscript and encouraged me to write a second book. Thanks to Skyhorse Publishing, who gave me a chance to show the world how healthy and delicious raw food is, and thanks to my editor Jenn McCartney and the Skyhorse team, who worked many hours to make this book look so beautiful.

I also want to thank all the new friends I met on this world journey who helped me understand their countries' food, spices, and culture: Chef Christine Mayr; Frank Capallades; Marie Tissot; Wendy C. Davis; Chef Kim Jansen; Chef Boris Lauser; Jean Jury of La Mano Verde; Dörte Bodenschatz; Karla Stereochemistry; Nick Eii; Donna Brown; Eduardo Salvia; Eraj Shakib; Vivi Letsou; George Cassimedes; the Guptas: Rakesh, Deepti, Krishna, Madhu, Smriti, Kunal, and Prarthna; Sunny and Yupin Riantawan; and Jennifer and Kevin Robertson. A big thank you to everyone who came to my speaking engagements on my world tour—you gave meaning to my trip, and I learned so much from all of you.

Last but not least, I thank my dear, sweet departed mother who always told me, "The way to a man's heart is through his stomach."

Index